What Women Need to Know

FROM HEADACHES TO
HEART DISEASE AND
EVERYTHING IN BETWEEN

For Emma Connolly Legato
December 26, 1913-April 3, 1996

Acknowledgments

We would like to acknowledge the unfailing, intelligent, and enthusiastic support of our editor, Laurie Bernstein, for the concept of this book. Without her we would not have completed the task. We would also like to thank the following physicians for sharing their expertise: David Bickers, M.D., chairman of the Department of Dermatology, Columbia Presbyterian Medical Center; Maria Bustillo, M.D., Mount Sinai Medical Center; Hiram Cody III, M.D., Memorial Sloan-Kettering Cancer Center; Alan M. Engler, M.D., New York plastic surgeon; Roy Geronemus, M.D., director of the Laser and Skin Surgery Center of New York; Fredi Kronenberg, M.D., director of the Richard and Hinda Rosenthal Center for Complementary and Alternative Medicine at the College of Physicians and Surgeons at Columbia University; Mary Gail Mercurio, M.D., Department of Dermatology, Columbia Presbyterian Medical Center; Harold Mermelstein, M.D., associate professor, New York University Medical School; and Richard Scher, M.D., Columbia Presbyterian Medical Center. A special thanks to Annie Hughes for all of her help during this and other projects.

Table of Contents

What Women Need to Know

Introduction

I am an internist with a private practice in New York City and a specialist in women's health. My colleagues and I have founded a center at
Columbia University College of Physicians & Surgeons that is dedi-
cated to improving doctors' understanding of the unique needs of
women patients.

In our first book, *The Female Heart: The Truth About Women and Coronary
Disease,* Carol and I shattered many myths about the health of women in general and about heart disease in particular. We alerted both women and their
physicians to the much ignored fact that cardiovascular disease is an equal
opportunity killer and the chief killer of American women. In fact, it claims
the lives of 500,000 women a year. (In contrast, fewer than 190,000 women
die each year from all cancers combined.) At the time we published *The
Female Heart,* many medical schools were still teaching that heart disease was
exclusively a plague of white males. We denounced this fallacy in our book
and talked about the astonishing prevalence of gender discrimination in
medicine. Up until then, women were excluded from most of the major medical studies, and little was known about how heart disease—or most other
diseases for that matter—affected women. As a result of this ignorance, the
legitimate complaints of women patients were often dismissed as hysterical
and not real. A woman with chest pains was sent home with a prescription

for Valium while a man with chest pains was sent to the nearest emergency room for further tests! Since *The Female Heart*, there have been some positive changes in the practice of medicine, but much more still needs to be done. That is why Carol and I are writing *What Every Woman Needs to Know: From Headaches to Heart Disease and Everything in Between*.

I've traveled widely throughout the United States over the last several years speaking to groups of women about health issues. I was astounded, at virtually every place I stopped—north and south, east and west, small towns and large cities—by the number of women who waited patiently to ask me questions after my talk. I was even more amazed by the types of questions they were asking me. They were rarely related to the topic of discussion but were, instead, about very basic worries they had about their health. Often the questions had to do with a peculiar symptom they were experiencing, or the side effects of medicines they were taking, or sexual issues they were confronting. But what I found most disconcerting was that these women were asking me—a total stranger—the kinds of questions they should have been asking their own doctors! After a while, I began to ask these women why they were asking me these questions, and why they felt they couldn't ask their own physicians. Their typical replies were most revealing:

"I didn't think it was important enough to bother him."
"The doctor was rushing through the examination and I didn't have time to ask."
"I was afraid she would think I was being silly."
"Frankly, I was afraid to hear the answer."
"I was too embarrassed to ask!"
"I didn't want her to think I was weird."
"It happened on the weekend, and I didn't want to disturb him."

These answers probably sound familiar to you, and some of them may even strike you as funny, and, of course, to an extent they are. But the bottom line is that the failure of women to communicate with their doctors can also be downright dangerous.

I acknowledge that doctors should shoulder much of the blame. All too often our waiting rooms are overcrowded, patient visits are rushed, and some of us even discourage the kind of personal conversation that will lead patients to feel comfortable enough to talk about what is really on their minds. But sometimes the problem rests on the other side of the desk or the examination table. Indeed, I've noticed that when a patient is particularly embarrassed or fearful about a topic, it emerges, if at all, only at the end of our "interview." For example, a woman I saw yesterday in my office confided, *after* I had talked to her for an hour and a half about her other, much less serious health concerns, that she had had five days of rectal bleeding. When I asked her why she hadn't mentioned such a serious symptom right away, she burst into tears, saying that she was afraid that, like her father, she was' going to die of colon cancer.

Although both men and women can feel rushed or neglected or too embarrassed to ask what they think is a "weird" question, the problem is often worse for women. For one thing, women know from experience that, in many cases, when they ask about a symptom or voice a concern, doctors are too quick to dismiss the problem as being "all in her head," whereas men with identical complaints are taken at their word, referred for further testing, or sent posthaste to the nearest emergency room! Moreover, I fear that in the new world of "managed care" medicine, in which time spent with a patient is often limited and treatment decisions are influenced significantly by financial considerations, this patient/doctor communication gap is bound to widen, and women patients are going to feel it first...and worst.

We have written this book to help close this communication gap. Our aim is not only to answer your pressing questions but also to teach and encourage you to speak up to your own doctor and ask all your questions in researching and writing this book, we have tried to identify the kinds of questions that weigh most heavily on women's minds—the kind that awaken us in the middle of the night in a cold sweat or distract us when we're trying to accomplish seventy-two hours worth of work in twenty-four. Some of these questions cause us to worry unnecessarily, but sometimes they really are matters of life and death. We have also taken pains to answer those questions women frequently feel are too trivial (or too "weird") to ask their own doctors but which in fact are vital to their health and well-being. In point of fact, I think *any* physical or emotional health issue that causes you concern, regardless of how silly or insignificant you may believe your doctor will think it is, is important and should be answered. Sometimes a simple answer will be all that's necessary to reassure you. In other cases, a seemingly insignificant question could turn out to be the most important one you will ever ask—and have answered.

HOW TO USE THIS BOOK

THIS BOOK IS organized alphabetically by subject, providing answers to questions ranging from cancer to menopause to skin care to yeast infections. Each entry includes the latest, up-to-date information on the best medical treatments for women. (A complete list of the subjects covered can be found in the contents, page 9.)

You can use this book:

- As *a resource* that will help you answer your questions before, after, and in between visits to your own doctor.
- As *a guide* to framing your questions so that your doctor will be able to understand and answer them. We can't make your doctor slow down or see fewer patients, but we can help you make the most effective use of your doctor's time (and your own). We will show you how to describe symptoms and troublesome issues so that your doctor can respond clearly and directly and provide the best possible advice.
- As *a reference* that will direct you to additional sources of information concerning a wide variety of health related issues. (We have included a comprehensive resource section, which begins on page 219.)

But perhaps the most important purpose of this book is to change your attitude about your own health and well-being. One of the most disturbing things I've learned in three decades of practicing medicine is that most of us women do not consider our own health needs to be as important as those of our loved ones. Ironically, many women can tell you in great detail about the ailments of their husbands or children, even of their parents or in-laws, but are oblivious of their own medical needs. I know women who can tell you their husbands' cholesterol levels (and when they were last checked) but who have never had their own cholesterol levels monitored. I've met countless women who insist that their husbands have annual physicals each year but who have never seen an internist themselves, and go to the gynecologist only when an obvious problem arises. Many women don't even have the most important screening tests done, such as a mammogram to detect breast cancer or a Pap smear to uncover cervical cancer. Such women—who wouldn't dream of letting their children miss an appointment with the orthodontist—are putting their lives at risk.

The bottom line is that women must be as concerned about their own health as they are about the health of their loved ones. We believe it is time for women to pick up the telephone and make some doctors' appointments on their own behalf, but even that is not enough. Our primary goal here is to give women the confidence they need to walk into their doctor's office ready and willing to get the information they need.

MARIANNE LEGATO, M.D.
January 1997

Abortion

Q. *I heard there is a new pill that can induce abortion so that a surgical abortion is no longer necessary. Is this true? Is it safe to use? Can I take it at home?*

A. There are two different types of drug therapies that can terminate preg-nancy; one is available in the United States and one is not. In my opinion, at this time, neither therapy is better than conventional surgical abortion.

RU 486, the so-called abortion pill, is widely used in France. When com-bined with oral prostaglandins (substances that cause the uterus to contract), RU 486 can induce abortion up to the ninth week of pregnancy. As of this writing, however, RU 486 is not legal in the United States; therefore, it is not an option for American women. Anti-abortion forces have so far been effec-tive in their efforts to block the use of RU 486 as an abortion drug, and it is only available in the United States to medical researchers for experimental purposes. Recent studies have suggested that RU 486 may be an effective treatment against breast cancer and other diseases, and a handful of American scientists are conducting further research.

There is another drug regimen for abortion that is both legal and available in the United States, but it is very new and somewhat controversial.

1

According to a study published in the *New England Journal of Medicine*, two other drugs commonly prescribed for other purposes can, when combined, also safely and effectively terminate pregnancy up to nine weeks. The first drug, methotrexate, is approved by the Food and Drug Administration (FDA) to treat some cancers as well as rheumatoid arthritis and psoriasis. The second drug, misoprostol, is an approved anti-ulcer medication that can also cause uterine contractions. For the past decade, methotrexate has been prescribed "off label" (not for its approved use) to terminate ectopic pregnancies (a potentially life-threatening condition that occurs when the fertilized egg lodges within the fallopian tube). Misoprostol is also commonly prescribed "off label" to soften the cervix when inducing labor.

In order to induce abortion, the patient must be given a shot of methotrexate, which terminates a pregnancy in two ways: It interferes with the growth of the embryo and the placenta by killing rapidly dividing cells, and it also blocks the action of folic acid, an important B vitamin that is critical to the normal growth and development of the embryo. Five to seven days later, the patient must return to the doctor for a vaginal suppository containing misoprostol. Typically, within two days after getting the suppository, the woman will begin to bleed and cramp, as she would with a miscarriage. In rare cases, the pregnancy may not terminate and a surgical abortion is required.

There are some advantages to this new abortion procedure over surgical abortions. For one thing, it can be performed in any doctor's office and does not necessitate a hospital stay or a visit to an abortion clinic, which many women may find upsetting (particularly if anti-abortion people are picketing outside). For another, unlike a surgical abortion, which is best performed at around six weeks, the drug-induced abortion can be performed as soon as the woman knows she is pregnant, which eliminates the days or weeks of waiting.

There are some disadvantages, however, to this procedure that women should be aware of. First, the drug-induced abortion takes considerably longer than the usual surgical procedure. During the first twelve weeks of pregnancy, abortion is usually done by vacuum aspiration, which takes between ten and fifteen minutes. In this procedure, the cervix (at the entrance of the uterus) is dilated and a blunt-tipped tube is placed in the uterus. The tube is connected to a small suction machine which draws out the contents of the uterus. A vacuum aspiration can be performed with either local or general anesthetic. In most cases, after an hour or two of rest, the woman can go home. Although there may be some residual bleeding for up to two weeks, the abortion is over quickly and efficiently. On the other hand, the drug-induced abortion can take up to two weeks before the abortion is finalized, which can be emotion-

2

ally wrenching for many women. In addition, if unprepared, many women may be very distressed by the amount of bleeding and cramping, although most of the women who have had this procedure find that the pain is easily controlled with medications. In addition, since neither methotrexate nor misoprostol have been approved by the FDA for use for abortion, some doctors may be reluctant to administer them for this purpose. As of now, I personally would not recommend this procedure until it has been tested further.

Q. *I had an early abortion when I was a teenager and my doctor said that everything went well. Now that I want to get pregnant, I'm having difficulty. I sometimes think that I'm being punished for the abortion. Could the abortion have caused my fertility problems?*

A. A legal abortion performed by a doctor under sterile, medical conditions rarely results in fertility problems. Keep in mind that about 15 percent of all couples have difficulty conceiving for any number of reasons. If you are concerned about infertility, you should not assume that the abortion was to blame, but you should consult a fertility specialist for a complete diagnostic workup.

It is true, however, that illegal abortions, typically performed under less than sanitary conditions, could cause problems that might make it difficult to conceive. For example, infection, a common complication of illegal abortions, could cause scarring in the Fallopian tubes, thus closing down the passages the sperm must pass through to reach and fertilize the egg. In rare cases, an illegal abortion could cause a more serious complication, like a perforated or torn uterus, which is a medical emergency that often requires a hysterectomy. Fortunately, since abortions are legal and done in medical settings, these complications rarely, if ever, occur.

Q. *I had an abortion over twenty-five years ago. Since then, I have had one child and am happily married. Although I know that I made the right decision at the time, I still feel very bad about the abortion. In fact, lately I have been waking up at night crying. Is this normal? I'm becoming menopausal, and wonder if I'm just being "over-emotional."*

A. I frequently see women who, having had an abortion many years earlier, apparently without any ill effect, suddenly and inexplicably begin to grieve about it years later. Often the grief surrounds the loss of reproductive ability, as in the case of menopause, or the death of a child, or some other severe blow that makes them believe they are being punished for their past "sin" of abortion. If the patient is really suffering, I usually refer her to a psychiatrist. Very often, simply talking about the issues that may have pro-

3

voked the reawakening of regret and guilt may be enough to bring the patient relief. If the obsession over the abortion continues, the psychiatrist may prescribe an antiobsessive or antidepressant medication like Prozac.

I do not believe there is such a thing as being "overemotional." However, I tell patients who feel unable to deal with their emotions, whether they be of unbearable internal pressure, grief, sorrow, or simply anxiety, to get help early. Check with your family doctor first: She probably knows you the best and can refer you to the appropriate consultant if you need psychiatric care or medication.

Acquired Immune Deficiency Syndrome (AIDS)

Q. I read that women are now at greater risk of getting AIDS than men, and when we do get it, it is a more serious form of the disease. Is this true?

A. At one time, AIDS was considered a disease that primarily afflicted gay men. We now know that this is simply not true, and, in fact, the fastest-growing method of transmission of the AIDS virus is through heterosexual contact. Today, more than 40,000 women in the United States have been diagnosed with AIDS, and depending on whose figures you believe, anywhere from 120,000 to 400,000 women are believed to be infected with HIV. AIDS is now the fourth leading cause of death of women between the ages of fifteen and forty-four.

Due to anatomical differences, women may be more likely to contract the HIV virus than men; in fact, women are twice as likely to get AIDS from a male partner than men are from a female partner. For one thing, semen contains greater quantities of HIV than do vaginal secretions, which makes unprotected vaginal intercourse riskier for women than for men. In addition, a vagina contains more surface area than a penis, so there is more of a chance that the virus will find a place within the vaginal wall or cervix

5

to infiltrate into the bloodstream. And since the semen remains in the vagina for several hours after intercourse, there is also more time for the virus to inoculate the bloodstream.

When women first began contracting AIDS, it was widely believed that they were not only harder hit by the disease, but that they actually died more quickly than men. In fact, statistics bear this out: Men who were diagnosed with AIDS live up to six times longer than women with the disease. Similar studies have also shown that African Americans with AIDS have a poorer prognosis than do whites. Perplexed by the starkly different prognoses of AIDS patients based on gender and race, researchers began to investigate whether there were any physical differences in women and African Americans that made them particularly vulnerable to the ravages of HIV. Recent studies, though, show that the disparity in survival rates have little to do with race and gender and everything to do with quality of care. In one study, for example, researchers found that patients who received drugs to prevent AIDS-related infections in the early stages of their disease had a higher survival rate than those who did not, regardless of gender or race, or any other factors. In other words, AIDS patients who had access to good quality health care fared better than those who did not. For whatever reason, women and African Americans with AIDS did not have the same access to health care as men.

It is also important to note that until recently, physicians knew very little about the progression of AIDS in women. Nearly all of the earlier studies had been performed on men, and there was little information about the way HIV affected women's bodies. For example, physicians were unaware that HIV could manifest itself in women in the form of an abnormal Pap smear, genital ulcers, or recurrent vaginal yeast infections. As a result of this ignorance, many women were diagnosed late, or never diagnosed at all, and therefore never received the medical treatment they so desperately needed. In 1993, based on new information, the Centers for Disease Control (CDC) expanded its definition of AIDS to include on their list of warning signs previously excluded conditions, including cervical cancer and other genital infections, and particularly stubborn, recurrent, or unusually virulent vaginal yeast infections.

Q. *Can you get AIDS from oral sex with a man? What about using sex toys like vibrators on each other? (I heard that was "safe" as long as you did not have intercourse.) How about open mouth kissing?*

A. AIDS is caused by the human immunodeficiency virus (HIV), which is transmitted in either of two ways:

6

1. through blood or blood products, such as a blood transfusion, or sharing a needle with an infected person
2. through the exchange of body fluids, such as semen or vaginal secretions during sexual activity.

Oral sex In women, the virus passes through the skin into the body through tiny tears or sores in the vagina, mouth, or rectum. Latex condoms offer good protection against HIV, especially when combined with the spermicide nonoxynol-9. It is definitely possible to get infected through oral sex if the man ejaculates into your mouth. Keep in mind that even the "pre cum," the drops of fluid that are discharged from the penis prior to ejaculation, can contain HIV. Therefore, it is advisable to insist that your partner use an unlubricated condom during oral sex.

Anal sex Anal sex can be particularly risky because the muscles that ring the rectal area do not stretch readily and as a result, when under pressure from an entering penis, can easily tear or break, thus allowing the virus to enter the bloodstream. If you practice anal sex, be particularly careful about using a condom and spermicide.

Sex toys Many people tell me that they are using so-called sex toys such as vibrators and dildos, particularly for anal sex, because they believe that the AIDS virus cannot be transmitted unless there is direct contact between the penis and the vagina, rectum, or mouth. Theoretically, the use of sex toys are safe if you use them on your partner and do not use the same toy on yourself. If, for example, a woman uses a vibrator on her partner, and then penetrates her vagina with the same vibrator, she could very well be infecting herself with HIV if her partner carries the virus.

As far as kissing is concerned, although HIV may be present in the saliva of infected individuals, it is not present in a high enough quantity to be considered a major threat. Blood-to-blood transmission of HIV from kissing may be possible if both people have open, bleeding sores. There was recently a reported case of AIDS being transmitted via a bite that penetrated the skin; however, the saliva was not the means of transmission. The person who did the biting had open sores in her mouth, which exposed the other to her blood.

Q. *I heard that lesbians do not get AIDS. Is this true?*

A. There is an extremely low incidence of AIDS among the lesbian population, which has led some people to believe that lesbians are somehow "immune" to

7

this disease. In reality, there has not been very much research done in this area, but based on what we do know, it appears as if lesbians would be as vulnerable as anyone else to contract HIV if they engage in risky behavior. Studies show that many lesbians are actually bisexual and may very well have sex with men as well as women. Some also use IV drugs. Since the AIDS virus can be transmitted through vaginal fluid, and even menstrual blood, it is very possible that AIDS can be transmitted by sexual contact between women.

Q. *When I was in college twelve years ago, I was not as careful as I should have been about sex. I was on the pill, and since I was not worried about pregnancy, I had sex with several partners without using a condom. I recently discovered that at least one of these individuals may have used heroin. Now that I am older and wiser, I'm worried that I may have contracted HIV. Should I be tested? What is the use of knowing you are HIV positive if AIDS is an incurable disease? I might add that I'm in perfect health. If I was HIV positive, wouldn't I be sick by now?*

A. Most people who contract the AIDS virus (HIV) begin to develop symptoms—so-called HIV disease—within eight to ten years of their initial exposure. HIV dampens the immune system's ability to work effectively. The role of the immune system is to fight against viruses and bacteria to prevent infection, and to identify potentially dangerous cells in the body that, if allowed to grow unfettered, could develop into cancer. In particular, HIV knocks out important cells called CD4, which are essential for the body to wage an effective battle against unwanted invaders. In time, HIV-infected women usually develop telltale symptoms of a compromised immune system, such as chronic and intractable yeast infections, severe respiratory infections, weight loss, skin rashes, night sweats, swollen glands, and cervical cancer. The Centers for Disease Control defines "full-blown" AIDS as the presence of two or more AIDS-related illnesses in persons who test positive for HIV.

If you have not had any of the symptoms listed above and you are in general good health, it is a good sign that you are not HIV positive; however, it does not guarantee that you are free of HIV. In rare cases, HIV disease may appear even later than ten years after the initial infection. In some cases, there are people who may test positive for HIV and remain perfectly healthy. According to a report in the New England Journal of Medicine (January 26, 1995), between 5 and 10 percent of HIV-infected people may not show any signs of the disease for a very long period of time, and it may even be possible that some may never develop full-blown AIDS. Researchers are studying these people to determine what, if anything, in their immune system is offering them special protection against the ravages of HIV.

8

I definitely think it is worthwhile for you to be tested for HIV, for several reasons. First, if you are not HIV positive, you can stop worrying needlessly. It takes up to six months to develop antibodies to HIV, which is a sign that you are infected. If you do not develop antibodies within six months of exposure, then you can rest assured that you are not HIV positive. Since your exposure was more than a decade ago, you will know for sure whether you have HIV by taking a simple blood test.

If you do test positive for HIV, it is important for you to know that even though AIDS itself is not yet curable, there have been tremendous strides made in recent years in terms of treating the diseases caused by the HIV infection. For example, in the early days of the AIDS epidemic, many patients died of a particularly aggressive form of pneumonia caused by Pneumocystis carinii (PCP). Today, we have excellent new drugs to keep PCP at bay, and as a result, there has been a dramatic increase in the survival rate of people who receive this treatment. Other studies have confirmed that HIV-infected people who get early medical treatment, and are vigilant about maintaining their health, fare significantly better than people who do not. As more and more breakthroughs are made in the treatment of AIDS, it is ever-more critical for HIV-positive people to sustain their health so that they will survive long enough to take advantage of these new treatments, and perhaps even be cured by medications we do not yet have but which may well develop as a result of ongoing research. To get the best treatment for HIV, I recommend that anyone who tests HIV positive should call the department of medicine of their nearest hospital or medical school and ask for the name of the infectious disease specialists treating AIDS. These physicians will be up-to-date on the latest and most effective treatments.

Who should be tested for HIV? If you fall into any of the following categories, testing for HIV is advisable:

- A woman who has had sexual contacts with sexually active partners who did not use a latex condom.
- An IV drug user, or anyone who has shared needles with others for any reason, including body piercing or at tattoo parlors.
- Health care workers who have been exposed to body fluids (blood and semen) of infected patients.
- Anyone who has had a blood transfusion between the years 1978 and 1985, before the blood supply was screened for HIV.

In particular, women who are pregnant and fear they may be HIV positive owe it to their babies to be tested. There is a 30 percent chance that the mother will pass the virus on to her baby either through exposure during

9

delivery or breast feeding. The good news is, if the mother takes the antiviral drug AZT during pregnancy, she can reduce the probability that her baby will be infected by as much as 70 percent.

Q. *I am a widow in my fifties who is seeing a wonderful man with whom I am interested in having a sexual relationship. He is divorced and I know he has had affairs with other women before meeting me. He is a fine person, and I am sure has been selective about his partners. Here is my question: I know that AIDS is a serious problem among kids, but do I really need to worry about having sex with a heterosexual, non-drug-using man who is absolutely normal?*

A. I often get asked this question in various forms from my patients who believe that, somehow, a "wonderful man" or a "fine person" cannot possibly be HIV-infected. In fact, women in their fifties are less likely than any other age group to demand that a sexual partner be tested for AIDS, or even believe that they can get AIDS from a new partner. Being middle-aged and "respectable" is no protection against AIDS. Even if you assume that your friend has been that selective in his partners, you cannot assume that all of his partners have been completely honest with him. Perhaps he thought he was having an exclusive relationship with a woman, but his partner had been unfaithful. Is it a chance you really want to take? The risks are high: AIDS is an incurable disease. The reality is: If a man or a woman is sexually active outside of a long-term, monogamous relationship, there is no guarantee that he or she is not infected with the AIDS virus. The only way to know conclusively that someone is "safe" is to insist on having yourself and your partner tested for HIV prior to embarking on an affair. Keep in mind that you must be tested six months after your last sexual contact to know for certain whether or not you are harboring the AIDS virus. If your partner refuses to be tested, it should raise a red flag, and I recommend that you proceed with great caution.

Alcohol

Q. *I have read that drinking a glass or two of wine a day can help prevent heart attacks. Is this true for women? I don't drink that much; should I start?*

A. You are referring to studies that have shown that women who drink one or two glasses of wine—or any kind of alcoholic beverage for that matter—have higher levels of HDL, "good cholesterol," which protects against heart disease. Since heart disease is the number-one killer of women, anything that can prevent this problem warrants serious consideration. Still, I don't think there's a responsible doctor on the planet who is going to advise a patient who does not drink to begin drinking. Whatever health benefits can be achieved from alcohol are quickly offset by the very real risks associated with problem drinking. Although the studies are inconclusive, women who drink heavily may be at greater risk of getting breast cancer than those who abstain. Heavy drinking is also associated with cirrhosis of the liver, which can be more severe in women. Even moderate drinkers may be at greater risk of getting osteoporosis, a disease that is characterized by the thinning of the bones.

Of special concern is the fact that incidence of solitary drinking among women is increasing, and especially among older women. In fact, the

American Medical Association (AMA) recently alerted physicians to the fact that alcohol abuse is on the rise in older patients who may use alcohol to cope with depression and loneliness.

Given the downside of alcohol, I believe that if you don't drink, there is no reason to start. If you do drink, do not exceed two glasses of alcohol a day. (A standard drink is defined as containing half an ounce of absolute alcohol. By this measure, the typical glass of wine is 4-5 ounces; a serving of hard liquor is about 1 ounce.)

There are some women who should not drink alcohol under any circumstances. Among them are women who are pregnant or who are trying to conceive (alcohol can cause severe birth defects), women who have had a history of problem drinking or who come from a family with a history of alcohol addiction, and women who are taking medication that could interact with alcohol.

Q. *A drink or two makes me feel sexy. Is this normal?*

A. Reactions to alcohol are as varied as the people who use it! Some women feel sexier and less inhibited after a few drinks, while others may feel shier and more withdrawn. Alcohol is a strong drug, and like any other drug, it will affect different people in different ways.

There is, however, some truth to the belief that alcohol can make women more receptive to sex. In the old days, gynecologists used to advise virgins to have a few drinks on their wedding night to prepare themselves for sex. Studies have shown that alcohol can reduce cortical control of behavior in some people, thereby lessening their ability to "censor" their behavior. We also know that alcohol can reduce anxiety in some drinkers, thus making sexual arousal more likely. Paradoxically, alcohol can also increase anxiety, especially in individuals with panic disorders.

Alcohol may also have an effect on hormones, the chemical messengers that control many bodily functions, including sexuality. A single study done by Finnish and Japanese investigators showed a rise in women's testosterone levels within two hours after drinking alcohol. Testosterone can stimulate libido in women, but it can also make some people aggressive, combative, and irritable (which is why some people become "mean drunks"). Whether or not this rise in testosterone is related to increased feelings of sexuality is difficult to say. People who drink alcohol often do so in settings where sexual encounters are possible, such as on dates or at home with a significant other. The increased sexual interest that you are experiencing could just as well be due to the relaxed setting, the company, and an expectation of a romantic encounter.

Q. *Does alcohol affect women differently than men?*

A. It definitely does. Women absorb alcohol faster than men, and so it takes less alcohol to make them drunk. We don't know precisely why this is so; however, it may be due to the fact that women do not produce as much of a key stomach enzyme—alcohol dehydrogenase—that is required to break down alcohol. In addition, women tend to be smaller than men; therefore, the same amount of alcohol is absorbed over less body surface. If you're going to drink, do so on a full stomach to slow down absorption rates.

Frequent exposure to high doses of alcohol can actually interfere with the normal production of the hormones that control the menstrual cycle. In fact, heavy drinkers often become menopausal earlier than social drinkers.

Q. *I work hard during the week and party hard on the weekends. I often have several glasses of beer and wine on a weekend night and have at times drunk so much that I pass out. I don't drink at all during the week. Is there anything wrong with an occasional binge?*

A. Whether you do it once a month or once a week, as far as I'm concerned, drinking until you pass out is a serious problem. Alcohol is a drug, and drinking to the point of unconsciousness is, in effect, a drug overdose. As I frequently remind my patients, in high enough doses, alcohol is a poison, and if blood-alcohol levels become too high, it can be lethal.

What I find particularly alarming about your drinking pattern is that you are putting yourself at risk in more ways than you can imagine. Alcohol can severely impair your judgment. Statistically, we know that women who are heavy drinkers are more likely to become victims of date rape and other forms of sexual assault. Even if you consent to sexual activity while under the influence, you will probably not have the clarity of thought to insist that your partner use a condom, which puts you at risk of pregnancy if you are not using another form of contraception and, even if you are, at risk of contracting a sexually transmitted disease such as herpes, AIDS, or chlamydia. If you are drunk, you are also more likely to get into a car with a driver who is intoxicated, and that, too, can be deadly.

From what you are telling me, weekend drinking appears to have become your way of dealing with the stress you're under during the week. You need to find a healthier and safer escape valve.

Q. *I am engaged to marry a man whose father and brother are problem drinkers. My fiancé does not drink at all, but I'm worried about our children. Is alcoholism genetic?*

A. There is no question that alcoholism is often clustered in families; both social and genetic factors figure into the cause of this devastating disease. I

13

have to be honest with you: The fact that two immediate relatives of your fiancé are problem drinkers is a concern. Even if he himself does not drink, your children may inherit a tendency to develop the disease. I am not going to advise you not to marry the man you love; however, you should go into this marriage knowledgeable about the potential pitfalls, and more important, you should take the necessary steps to avoid them.

I strongly advise you and your future husband to get some professional counseling about alcoholism so that you are both aware of the risks. Since you know that your children stand a chance of inheriting a predisposition for alcoholism, it is imperative for them to be counseled about their susceptibility, on the basis of genetics, to alcoholism. In this situation, forewarned is forearmed.

Here are some other facts you should know:

- The two major risk factors for alcoholism are male sex and a family history of alcoholism.
- More alcoholics are men: They have a lifetime risk of a 3-5 percent chance of becoming dependent on alcohol compared with women, in whom there is a 1 percent lifetime risk.
- When male sex and a positive family history both exist, the risk is highest; 25 percent of the sons of alcoholic fathers become alcoholics themselves.

These things "cluster" (the likelihood of coexisting and related characteristics): male gender, early onset of problem drinking, familial alcoholism, a serious dependence on alcohol, a more rapidly deteriorating course, and a greater likelihood of alcohol-related problems (like criminal behavior).

Q. *What's the best way to deal with a hangover from excessive drinking?*

A. An alcohol hangover can cause a painful headache as well as a sick, woozy feeling. Fortunately, a hangover usually does not last for more than a day, but it can be a day of sheer hell. There are several things you can do to reduce the pain and discomfort. First, an ice pack applied to your head will relieve the pain of a throbbing headache. Caffeine, found in coffee and tea, will constrict the blood vessels in your head, which will also help relieve some of the pain. In fact, the best hangover cure of all may be a cup or two of strong tea with honey. According to the National Institute of Neurological and Communicative Disorders and Stroke, honey speeds up alcohol metabolism, which means that it will help your body break down the alcohol more quickly.

I do not recommend nonsteroidal anti-inflammatory drugs such as ibuprofen or Naprosyn, since these drugs can irritate the stomach lining which may already be irritated from the alcohol, and could even cause bleeding. Instead, use Alka-Seltzer, which is easier on the stomach and contains a combination of aspirin (combats headache), sodium bicarbonate (neutralizes excess stomach acid), and citric acid (reduces nausea). Do not take excessive amounts of acetaminophen (Tylenol) after consuming alcohol. The combination of alcohol and acetaminophen can produce kidney damage, especially on an empty stomach, which can be lethal.

Prescription headache drugs such as ergotamine, which is used to treat migraine headaches, have also been shown to cure the hangover headache. If you happen to have a prescription headache drug on hand, ask your doctor if you can take it for a hangover. Part of the discomfort of a hangover is from a state of dehydration and electrolyte depletion, so try to drink plenty of liquids, especially those like consommé, which have salt or to which you can add salt. Contrary to popular belief, a shot of alcohol does not "cure" a hangover; it will only make you feel sicker.

Alzheimer's Disease

Q. *Since I have become menopausal, I have become very forgetful. Although I have no trouble remembering events that happened a long time ago, I do have difficulty recalling such simple things as the name of a person to whom I was just introduced. Am I showing signs of Alzheimer's disease?*

A. Loss of memory for names is extremely common in both sexes after the age of forty and is a normal phenomenon of aging. It is not unusual that you would begin to notice these memory lapses after menopause; as I discuss in the next question, estrogen plays a role in brain function, and the decline in estrogen could affect memory.

Symptoms of Alzheimer's disease go far beyond that of forgetting names or even important dates. Alzheimer's is characterized by a myriad of other problems including the inability to communicate, sudden mood changes, confusion, irrational behavior, and the inability to cope with daily living. Unless you are experiencing some of these other symptoms, I would not worry about your memory loss.

There are some things you can do to help improve your memory function. Many women find that taking hormone replacement therapy (HRT) after menopause helps restore memory and even improves the ability to concentrate. I do not take estrogen myself, but I rely on "mind games" to help me remember names. Specifically, I try to make an association with the name that will stick in my mind. For example, I was recently introduced to a woman named Rita who, like the actress Rita Hayworth, had red hair. In my mental file, I stored "red hair" with "Rita Hayworth." The next time I met this woman, I was able to retrieve her name. This technique works well for many people. I also find it helpful to use the name of the person in conversation immediately after being introduced; this also helps to reinforce the name in your mind.

Q. *I read that estrogen can prevent Alzheimer's disease, which is of special interest to me since my grandmother had Alzheimer's, and I would like to avoid the kind of mental and physical deterioration that she experienced. Should I take estrogen replacement therapy after menopause? Why would a sex hormone affect mental function?*

A. Although it has not yet been proven, there appears to be a link between lack of estrogen and Alzheimer's disease, a degenerative disease characterized by memory loss, mood changes, and physical deterioration. Interestingly, there also appears to be a connection between estrogen levels and mental functioning in healthy women.

After menopause, estrogen levels drop precipitously as ovarian function begins to wane and menstruation stops. There are many other changes that occur as we age, and one of the most dramatic is a loss in short-term memory. Typically, it becomes more difficult to recall the names of new acquaintances or to absorb new facts. Some researchers suspect that the lower levels of estrogen may somehow affect the ability to remember. Several studies have shown that postmenopausal women who are on hormone replacement therapy—HRT—(estrogen and progesterone) score better on memory tests than women who are not taking hormones. For example, researchers at Stanford University studied 144 women between the ages of fifty-five and ninety-three, half of whom were taking estrogen and half who were not. Each woman was asked to look at photographs of six male and six female faces with a common first and last name. They were given one minute to study each picture. The women were later shown the pictures of the faces and asked to write down the corresponding name. The women on HRT did markedly better, getting 36 percent of the names right, versus a correction rate of only 26 percent for the group not taking hormones. For doctors like myself who have been prescribing estrogen to patients, the results of this study came as no surprise. Indeed, many women claim that they not only feel better taking HRT but that they actually can think better.

17

What is even more intriguing are studies that have shown that young women do better on memory tests when they are in the high phase of their estrogen cycle (the first half) than when they are in the low phase—during menstruation. In other words, if these studies are correct, even the normal monthly fluctuations of estrogen can affect a woman's ability to remember.

Estrogen may not only improve memory but, more important, it may also protect against Alzheimer's disease. In one groundbreaking study at the University of Southern California, researchers have been tracking, since 1981, 8,877 women residents in a Los Angeles retirement community. By 1992, 2,529 of these women had died. Out of the deceased group, 138 had Alzheimer's or some form of dementia listed on their death certificate. The researchers then reviewed each woman's medical history, in particular checking to see whether she had had HRT. The researchers found that women on HRT were much less likely to develop Alzheimer's than women who were not taking hormones. In fact, the researchers calculated that women on HRT are 30 percent less likely to get Alzheimer's. Based on this study, it would appear that taking HRT can reduce the risk of Alzheimer's disease, although, the researchers themselves caution that more studies are needed before there can be a definitive conclusion drawn regarding the ability of estrogen (HRT) to protect against Alzheimer's.

Clearly, estrogen plays some kind of role in helping us to think, recall facts, and preserve mental function. Although estrogen is best known for its role in reproduction, it is not just confined to the reproductive system; in fact, it is used by cells throughout the body, even in the brain. Studies have shown that estrogen can actually increase the number of processes or projections on nerve cells (called dendrites) in the brain that are involved in memory, and Alzheimer's patients have a severe deficit of these important processes. The ability to promote the formation of dendrites may be why estrogen helps to prevent Alzheimer's disease. Another interesting fact: In rats, estrogen increases the amount of acetylcholine, a chemical in the brain called a neurotransmitter that is also involved in memory. Whether this is also true in humans remains to be seen.

To answer your original question, should you take estrogen to protect yourself against Alzheimer's depends on many factors, including whether you are a good candidate for HRT. (For more detailed information on HRT, see the questions on menopause.)

Anemia

Q. *I've been feeling tired. I think I may be anemic. Should I take iron pills?*

A. Not until you know for sure you are anemic and what type of anemia you have.

Anemia is a fairly common problem among adolescent girls and women who are still menstruating. To most people, anemia is simply another word for "iron deficiency," and they think that taking a few iron pills will solve the problem. Anemia is actually a complex disorder and may be caused by a number of different factors, some serious, some not. In most cases, a patient may not even know she has a mild anemia until it is discovered on a routine blood test called a CBC, or complete blood count. In some cases, however, a patient may feel so exhausted and fatigued that she seeks help from her doctor.

Anemia is a problem that results when the cells of the body are not getting enough oxygen. Living tissue needs oxygen; it "breathes," or to use the scientific term, it "respires." Respiration is the process in which cells perform a series of chemical reactions, all of which require oxygen, to make enough energy to function and maintain themselves. When we are anemic, our cells are deprived of oxygen. Anemia can be due to one of two things: not enough of a compound called hemoglobin, which carries oxygen in the blood; or not enough red blood cells, the special cells in which hemoglobin is packaged and carried throughout the bloodstream. When oxygen supplies fall to critically low levels, tissue can actually die, and vital organs like the heart and brain can be permanently impaired. People with even partial obstruction of blood vessels due to arteriosclerosis—who are not getting enough oxygen to their vital organs to begin with—can be seriously impacted by anemia, which can even result in a heart attack.

If a woman is anemic, her physician will first try to determine the cause of the anemia. There are several possibilities:

Iron deficiency Since iron is needed to produce hemoglobin, a lack of hemoglobin is often a sign of iron deficiency. Women who have heavy menstrual periods or who do not eat iron-rich foods are at risk of developing an iron deficiency.

Not enough B vitamins Folic acid and vitamin B12, both forms of vitamin B, are essential for the production of the red blood cells that carry the hemoglobin. A diet deficient in either of these vitamins could result in too few red blood cells, which could cause anemia. In fact, many older people suffer from a vitamin B12 deficiency because of a lack of gastric acid, which is needed to break down protein, an important source of B12.

Abnormal hemoglobin In some cases, the structure of the hemoglobin molecule is abnormal so that the process of oxygen delivery and release is adversely affected, thus causing anemia. This is precisely what happens in the case of sickle cell anemia, a disease that primarily affects African Americans.

Bone marrow failure Cells needed to make red blood cells are produced in the bone marrow; however, in some cases, a defect in bone marrow could result in a depression of the production of these key cells, thus resulting in anemia. In fact, some medications, including many anticancer drugs, can thwart the production of bone marrow cells.

Destruction of red blood cells An overactive spleen or a defect in the red blood cells themselves can lower the total red blood cell count to an unsafe level.

Excess blood loss Anemia may be the first sign of a problem such as colon cancer where the loss of blood may be steady, severe, and silent.

TREATMENT

DO NOT SELF-MEDICATE. If you are diagnosed with anemia, do not assume that popping an iron supplement will cure the problem. (In some cases, taking iron when you don't need it can cause an even greater problem, see page 141.) Be sure that your physician knows not only how anemic you are but what is causing the problem.

For most women, however, treatment is quite simple. If iron stores are deficient, eating more iron-rich foods (such as red meat, liver, tuna, turkey) and taking an iron supplement will help relieve the problem. Many fruits and vegetables also contain iron, but it's in a form that is not as easily absorbed by the body. The absorption of this so-called non heme iron can be greatly improved by taking a vitamin C supplement.

If your physician discovers that a lack of folic acid or vitamin B12 is the culprit, she can prescribe folic acid supplements or give you injections of vitamin B12, both of which will quickly correct the situation.

For those patients in whom the problem is due to blood loss, finding and correcting the source of the bleeding is crucial. Many menstruating women who have an excessive flow each month may have to take iron pills, as in the case of patients who have fibroid tumors. Blood transfusions are rarely needed except in extreme cases, as can occur when an individual is in an accident and loses a critical amount of blood over a very short period of time. Most physicians will wait to transfuse until levels of red blood cells and/or hemoglobin are really quite low and there is not enough time for new cells and hemoglobin molecules to be formed to replete exhausted supplies.

Asthma

Q. *I have asthma, which makes it hard for me to breathe when I'm upset. My husband says it's psychosomatic and that I could control my asthma attacks if I wanted to. Is he right?*

A. An asthma attack occurs when the air tubes of the lungs become constricted, which can affect breathing. The symptoms of asthma are very real—they are not "in your head," nor are they under your control. There's no question, however, that emotional excitement—either extreme happiness or extreme upset—can produce an asthma attack in some individuals. In fact, half of all asthma patients experience a sense of constriction in the chest when they're excited. Why? When you're upset, the muscles around some parts of the breathing tube can squeeze down and release histamines into the respiratory tree, which can cause swelling, inflammation, and further obstruction of the airways. This is followed by a sense of shortness of breath or difficulty in breathing, coughing, and wheezing. The reason for this reaction is very complex and not fully understood. It is likely, however, that strong emotions may stimulate the autonomic nervous system that controls such automatic functions as the beating of our hearts, blood pressure, and breathing.

22

Taking your medications before you expect an upsetting time is a good idea: Use them if you are anticipating a confrontation with your husband about something, for example. Letting asthma stack the cards against a complete and fair discussion takes an unfair advantage and, in the long run, may postpone a real solution to your problem.

Bad Breath

Q. *I have a new boyfriend and a new problem—bad breath. Recently, much to my embarrassment, my boyfriend commented that my breath was bad, and suggested that I see a dentist. My dentist told me that my teeth are fine, but my breath still isn't. I brush regularly and use mouthwash, what more can I do?*

A. Bad breath is such a common complaint that there are actually breath clinics springing up around the country that specialize in treating this problem. In fact, it has been estimated that about 25 million Americans have a problem with bad breath at some point in their lives.

Bad breath is a result of the accumulation of anaerobic bacteria in the mouth, teeth, or gums that can emit unpleasant sulfur fumes. This particular breed of bacteria thrive in warm, dark places, and live on plaque deposits in teeth and food debris that may linger in the mouth or on the tongue. Gum disease or tooth decay is a leading cause of bad breath, and your boyfriend was correct to suggest that you see a dentist. Bad breath may also be a result of the monthly hormonal changes women go through. At the beginning of menstruation and during ovulation, women produce more protein in their saliva, which creates more sulfur fumes.

24

Based on what you are telling me, however, I suspect your breath problem may be caused by a decrease in saliva production due to stress. Saliva helps keep your breath fresh by constantly irrigating or washing out the mouth. Chronic stress can hamper the production of saliva, thus promoting bad breath. Now that you are embarking on a new romance, you may be feeling more anxious than normal, and this may be affecting your saliva flow. There are several things you can do to increase your saliva production and keep your breath fresh:

- Replace lost moisture: You will need to compensate for the decrease in saliva production by keeping your mouth moist. Try taking frequent sips of water throughout the day. Simple measures, such as sucking on sugar-free mints, may also help stimulate saliva flow and freshen your mouth.
- Use mouthwash: When the people at *Consumer Reports* tested popular brands of mouthwash, they found that most did freshen breath and eliminate odor, but within ten minutes to an hour they stopped working. Some of the new mouthwashes on the market, however, contain a compound called chlorine dioxide, which, according to several studies, may be more effective in controlling bad breath than some of the older mouthwashes.
- Clean your tongue: Although the tongue appears to be a smooth, slippery surface, it is actually loaded with crevices that can be a magnet for bacteria. Some dentists recommend that when you brush your teeth, you should also lightly brush your tongue. Interestingly, in Indian and Arab cultures, people use small shovel-like tongue scrapers several times a day to keep their breath fresh. Although tongue scrapers are sold in Middle Eastern and Indian markets, I recommend that you get one from a dentist who can show you the correct way to use it.

If these simple measures don't help your breath problem, your physician may prescribe a medication called pilocarpine (sold as Salogen) to help improve salivary flow. Pilocarpine works well for many people but should not be used by individuals with certain medical problems.

If your breath problem persists or gets worse, you should see your doctor. Bad breath is not just embarrassing; it could be a sign of a health problem. In addition to chronic stress, there are several other conditions that can be causing your bad breath, including a throat or sinus infection. If you have a chronic stuffy nose or a post-nasal drip, check with your physician to see if you have an infection. Very often, a course of antibiotics can clear up both the infection and the bad breath. In addition, some common physical ailments can cause a decrease in saliva flow, which will result in bad breath. For example, Sjögren's syndrome, an autoimmune disease that primarily strikes women, can cause chronic dry mouth. Very often, people with Sjögren's have other symptoms, including dry eye and joint pain. Certain medications, such as antidepressants and antihistamines, can also reduce salivary flow and cause bad breath. If it's medication that is causing your problem, your physician may be able to prescribe another one.

Blood Transfusions

Q. *I am scheduled to have a cesarean section next month and am very worried about the prospect of needing a blood transfusion during or after the operation. Is the blood supply safe? Should I donate my own blood? Can I refuse a transfusion if its not a life-threatening situation?*

A. Anytime I recommend surgery for one of my patients, I know one of the very next questions I will hear is, "If I need a blood transfusion, am I putting myself at risk of getting AIDS?" I put my patients' fears to rest by telling them the truth: Despite the widely publicized cases of people who have contracted HIV through blood transfusions, the reality is that the blood supply is probably safer than it has ever been.

Just ten years ago, technicians tested blood for only one contaminant: syphilis. Today, blood is screened for nine infectious agents in all, including HIV, the virus that causes AIDS, and hepatitis, a liver infection that can be fatal. Since 1985, when scientists realized that transfusions could transmit HIV infection, the Food and Drug Administration (FDA) introduced rigorous rules for blood banks. The FDA now monitors every step of the preparation process, beginning with donor screening and ending with the delivery of blood products to their destinations. As a result of this meticulous screening

27

process, there have been only twenty-nine reported cases of AIDS resulting from transfusions over the past nine years. This is an amazing statistic considering that 3.6 million people get transfusions of whole blood or blood products annually in the United States.

This is not to say, however, that getting a blood transfusion is risk-free. The test for HIV is not infallible; in fact, it can only detect HIV antibodies, which may take up to twenty-five days to be produced by the body after the person is infected. If an infected individual donates blood before the antibodies are produced, the test will not detect HIV, and the blood may be deemed safe. Due to this glitch in the testing process, there is a small but real risk that about 1 in 250,000 units of blood reaching patients will be infected with HIV. In addition, about 1 in 250,000 units of blood will harbor the hepatitis B virus, and 1 in 3,300 the hepatitis C virus. More often than not, the real risk of transfusion is human error. Statistically, transfusions carry about a 1 percent risk of some unanticipated outcome, ranging from contracting a serious infection to death. Studies show that mistakes in collecting, processing, or transfusing blood are much more frequent than infections. One of the most common mistakes is the administration of the wrong blood type, which in rare circumstances can be fatal. In most cases, however, doctors can handle most transfusion reactions quickly and effectively with antihistamines that block any adverse reactions to foreign blood proteins.

Given the fact that there is a real, albeit small, risk of developing a problem from a blood transfusion, here are my recommendations to minimize the risk:

Donate your own ahead of time Up to two weeks before surgery, you can bank your own blood. If you are pregnant, check with your doctor; anemia is a common problem in pregnancy and may make blood loss even for a later transfusion unwise.

Do not pressure your family or friends to donate blood Studies show that blood donations from friends and family are more likely to be infected with HIV or hepatitis than the blood from the blood banks. We do not know why this occurs; it may be due to the fact that family and friends who know they have a problem and normally would not donate to a blood bank may be more reluctant or embarrassed to refuse a friend or relative.

Ask about alternatives For many patients, there are safe alternatives to whole-blood transfusion, depending on what part of the blood is needed. For example, some people may need only one of the many proteins found in blood, and it may be possible to isolate this protein and deliver it for transfusion, thus reducing the volume of fluid delivered to the body, thereby reducing the risk of contracting an infection. There are even some drugs available today that can stimulate the patient's bone marrow to produce its own blood cells, thus eliminating the need for transfusion. Before surgery, be sure to talk to your physician about other options.

"Is this transfusion necessary?" Prior to the AIDS scare, many physicians would routinely order a blood transfusion after surgery to treat anemia and other conditions that are not life-threatening. Today, many physicians and patients resist blood transfusions unless a patient has lost a critical amount of blood. If your doctor does suggest a transfusion, you or a family member must make it clear that you will agree to have a transfusion only if it is absolutely essential, and not simply because it will speed up your recovery period.

Insist on close monitoring during the transfusion If you do need a transfusion, insist that you be monitored by a technician for at least fifteen minutes after the infusion begins to make sure you are tolerating the blood. If you are monitored and have a bad reaction, the technician can immediately discontinue the infusion and administer the appropriate treatment.

Get follow-up testing in two weeks If you have had a transfusion, ask your doctor to test you for hepatitis B within two weeks of the transfusion. If you have contracted this virus, early treatment can improve the prognosis for full recovery.

Body Image

Q. *I am not overweight, but I hate my body (I have heavy hips and thighs) and dread wearing a bathing suit or walking around in shorts. What can I do to (1) lose the fat where I want to lose it, and (2) learn to like myself better?*

A. For many women, physical appearance is inextricably linked to self-esteem, and when a woman is not happy with her body, she is often unhappy with herself. From a physician's perspective, one of the most serious problems for women is the fact that our culture emphasizes extreme youth and thinness as the criteria for feminine beauty. And ironically, the ideal for feminine beauty that is being promoted today is neither feminine nor particularly healthy. If you thumb through any of the fashion magazines you'll see pages of unrealistic (and unhealthy) images of painfully thin, androgynous models with bodies that have little resemblance to that of real women. Very few have decent muscle development or muscle tone: Instead of the smoothly sculpted backs of healthy women, their rear view is literally one of "skin and bones." I recently attended a fashion show, and I was alarmed by the pathologic thinness and even malnutrition of the models. I had to fight the impulse to invite them to my office for treatment!

What do real women look like? Most women tend to deposit fat on their hips and buttocks (the so-called gynecoid distribution of fat). The female distribution of fat is actually beneficial to your health because it protects against heart disease (it is better to carry fat around your hips than in the stomach) and serves as an important storage depot for estrogen after menopause. Take consolation in knowing that women who are too thin do not age as well as normal-weight women (wrinkles are often more obvious on taut skin), and they are prone to such estrogen-deprivation diseases as osteoporosis.

If a woman hates her body, I think she first needs to try to understand the source of these negative feelings, and more important, she needs to devise strategies to overcome them. Too many women—especially young ones—fall prey to this form of self-loathing. At times, it can even be fatal. As many as 5 percent of all young women have serious eating disorders—that is, they are quite literally starving themselves to achieve some unrealistic standard of thinness. Countless others go from diet to diet in a futile attempt to achieve the media's version of the perfect woman. It is essential to understand that there is no one correct standard of beauty; there must be room for many variations on the same theme.

The woman who hates her body also needs to do things that will make her feel better about herself. For many women, sculpting the body and toning flabby muscles can make a big difference in their self-image. For example, in one study, middle-aged women who felt that gravity was taking over their body contour had a much improved body image after a regimen of light weight lifting three times a week. Although none of the women lost any weight, they looked and felt better. Regular visits to a gym can do wonders for both your physique and your psyche.

31

Body Perspiration

Q. *I sweat so much that I know my clothes have a limited life. Furthermore, even the cleaner can't get out the stale smell this leaves. Why does this happen?*

A. There are many reasons for excessive underarm perspiration, one of which is anxiety, particularly in young women. Often, sweat literally pours down their arms and the sides of their chest when they have to speak in public, or when talking with someone with whom they are shy or uneasy. Simply getting into your thirties can solve most of this problem.

If sweating is destroying your clothes, try wearing cotton or another washable material next to your body. If you can't wash it right away, soak the garment as soon as possible after taking it off. Sweat itself doesn't smell offensive: It is the bacteria that grow in the area that cause the odor. Find a deodorant that cuts down problem sweating: Mitchum is a good one, but may cause underarm eruptions or burns in susceptible people.

Some illnesses cause excessive sweating; tuberculosis is one. Other excessive sweating results from alcoholism; as the alcohol wears off and withdrawal symptoms begin, perspiration increases. Sweat is a good growth medium for bacteria and explains why skin infections are more common in alcoholics than in the rest of the population.

Breasts

Q. *While browsing through a bookstore, I came across a book that claimed that underwire bras can cause breast cancer. I wear an underwire bra; am I increasing my risk of cancer?*

A. I searched the medical literature for studies on underwire bras and a possible link to cancer, and I did not find any. I also consulted with Dr. Hiram Cody III, an attending surgeon on the breast service at New York's Memorial Sloan-Kettering, one of the premier cancer treatment centers in the world. Dr. Cody, who says that he is frequently asked this question by his patients, confirms that there are absolutely no data to support the connection between the type of bra a woman wears and her risk of developing breast cancer. In Dr. Cody's own words, "Cancer is a complicated process. It's probably absurd to think that a bra has anything to do with it."

As to whether underwire bras are dangerous in other ways, I would have to say that there is a remote possibility that a poorly fitted or a worn-out bra could cause problems. For example, if a bra is too tight, it could cause significant pain due to pressure on the ribs. In addition, if the underwire supporting the cup breaks through the fabric and cuts the skin, it could in rare circumstances result in an infection. My advice is to use your common sense.

Do not wear a bra if it is too tight. If you wear an underwire bra, examine it carefully before each wearing. If the wire is beginning to poke through the fabric, retire the bra.

Q. *During my annual checkup, my gynecologist told me that I had fibrocystic breast disease. Although my doctor said it was no cause for concern, I'm worried. What should I know about this problem? Is there a cure? Am I more likely to get breast cancer?*

A. Fibrocystic breast disease is a fancy way of saying that you have lumpy breasts; it is a vague, general diagnosis that applies to many different conditions that are most often benign. I do not like using the term *fibrocystic breast disease* because it can unduly alarm patients and make them think something is abnormal when, in fact, it is not. Even a perfectly normal breast may have nodules that make it feel somewhat lumpy, particularly before or during your period. In fact, studies show that up to half of all women develop fibrocystic breasts at some time during their lives and that these mysterious "lumps and bumps" often disappear after menopause. These lumps are harmless; there is no evidence that fibrocystic lumps increase the risk of developing breast cancer.

How do doctors distinguish between a benign lump and one that is potentially malignant? A skilled practitioner can often determine the type of breast lump simply by feeling it; if your doctor thought you had a potentially serious problem, she undoubtedly would have suggested follow-up tests, including a mammogram or a sonogram, or even a biopsy. The fact that she did not order further testing means that your particular type of lumps felt normal.

There are many different types of benign breast lumps.

Cysts These are fluid-filled balloon-like sacs that have very distinct borders. Often, they feel more elastic and pliable than a solid mass. Usually, if a doctor feels a mass that she suspects is a cyst, she may ask you to return for another examination. Hormonal changes that occur before menstruation could cause breast cysts to retain fluid, which would disappear on its own after menstruation. Your doctor may also order an ultrasound examination to verify that the lump is indeed a fluid-filled cyst and not a solid mass. In some cases, the doctor may want to aspirate the cyst to determine if it is solid or filled with fluid. An aspiration is a simple procedure that involves removing fluid through a hollow needle. Some doctors offer their patients a shot of novocaine to relieve the pain, although many patients feel that the novocaine shot itself is so painful that they might as well just have the procedure without it. Usually, once it is aspirated, the cyst collapses and disappears, but if the fluid is bloody or rapidly reaccumulates, further investigation is

34

required. This usually means a breast biopsy, where the tissue can be examined under a microscope and tested for malignant characteristics.

Fibroadenoma Solid lumps can be benign collections of cells called a fibroadenoma; these lumps are typically described as having a "marblelike smoothness" and a rather slippery quality. Fibroadenoma occur most often in women under the age of thirty and tend to recur. In some cases, only a biopsy can determine whether this type of lump is malignant. Very often, doctors recommend the fibroadenoma be removed because it can grow and cause discomfort, primarily during pregnancy and lactation.

Intraductal papilloma These small, wartlike growths in the milk ducts can produce bleeding in the nipples.

Lipoma Lipomas are single, painless lumps that are usually found in postmenopausal women. These are perfectly round, soft, and somewhat movable.

Q. *Does caffeine cause "lumpy breasts"?*

A. There have been many anecdotal reports that link caffeine consumption to fibrocystic breasts, but there are no scientific studies to confirm this link. A handful of studies, however, have claimed that women with fibrocystic breasts who refrain from caffeine report a lessening in the severity of their symptoms. If you have fibrocystic breasts, you can try to cut down or even eliminate your intake of caffeine to see if it helps relieve any of your symptoms. Beware of hidden sources of caffeine: Although primarily known as an ingredient in coffee and tea, caffeine is also present in high quantities in colas, chocolate, and many over-the-counter analgesics.

Q. *Is it dangerous to pluck the hairs around the nipples? Can it cause breast cancer?*

A. There is absolutely no evidence that plucking hairs around the nipples is dangerous in any way. I would not, however, recommend waxing hair in this area because it could promote infection.

Q. *Every time I examine my own breasts I come across some lump or bump that I think is important, but when I see my doctor, he tells me it's normal. In light of my experience, is breast examination useful?*

A. There has been a great deal of emphasis in recent years placed upon the importance of self-examination of the breasts as a means of early detection of breast cancer. Not all breast specialists, however, feel that self-examination is effective, and in fact, many feel its importance has been overemphasized. For example, in her book *Dr. Susan Love's Breast Book*, the renowned breast specialist cautioned that urging women to perform self-examination of their breasts may not only promote undue anxiety, but may be expecting too much of patients. She added that expecting women to find their own breast cancer is tantamount to "blaming the victim" and relieving the medical establishment of their responsibility to find better diagnostic techniques. Dr. Love has a point. For one thing, a normal breast can feel lumpy, and only a skilled physician can distinguish between normal lumps and bumps and those that are abnormal. For another thing, in some women, self-examination can cause so much stress and unnecessary fear that it is far better for them to visit a doctor at appropriate intervals than to continue to make themselves nervous wrecks.

This is not to say that self-examination is a worthless exercise—not at all. It can be an important tool for the detection of cancer. In fact, 90 percent of all breast lumps are first discovered by the women themselves, and although about 80 percent of these lumps are not malignant, there are cases in which women owe their lives to their own self-examination. Nevertheless, studies have not shown that self-examination improves breast cancer mortality since many cancers that are asymptomatic and easy to feel are simply of the slow-growing and less-lethal type. In my opinion and in the opinion of most breast specialists, regular mammography combined with a careful examination by an experienced physician remains the most effective and accurate way to detect breast cancer: Together they detect over 95 percent of malignancies.

Q. *Is there any connection between diet and breast cancer?*

A. It has been very hard to either prove or disprove a positive link between diet and an increased risk of breast cancer primarily because there have been few serious studies on this subject. Research funded by the Women's Health Initiative is under way, but it will be more than a decade before these studies will yield any definitive results. Even though there is no concrete evidence linking diet to breast cancer, there are some convincing arguments. The fat connection: One of the more controversial issues in medicine is whether a diet high in fat increases the risk of breast cancer. Many experts argue that it does, and there is at least circumstantial evidence to support this claim. The rates of breast cancer are substantially higher in the West where the fat intake is the highest, and much lower in Asia and Africa where the fat intake is the lowest. For example, in the United States, Americans consume about 36 percent of their daily calories as fat, much of it in the form of saturated fat, which is found in meat and dairy, and transfatty acid, which is found in margarine.

In contrast, in many Asian countries, the daily intake of fat is under 15 percent of daily calories, and the cuisine is primarily vegetarian. Could a high-fat diet be the reason why an American woman has four times the chance of dying from breast cancer than a Japanese woman? Could diet explain another enigma: When Japanese women move to the United States, within one generation their risk of dying from breast cancer is equal to that of other Americans. It is hard to deny that environmental factors, including diet, play some role in breast cancer.

A handful of studies have also shown a connection between a high-fat diet and midline obesity (bulging abdomen), which we know is a risk factor for breast cancer. Yet a major study of thousands of nurses showed that there was little difference in the fat intake of women who had developed breast cancer and women who did not. Critics of this study contend that all the nurses in the study were on diets relatively high in fat—most consuming more than 30 percent of their daily calories as fat—and that comparing one high-fat diet to another was meaningless. They argue that in order to do a study effectively, you need to compare the fat intake of women on low-fat diets (under 20 percent) to those on the typical American high-fat diet.

To add to the confusion, other studies suggest that fat per se is not the enemy; it is the *kind* of fat you eat that's important. For example, although women in Mediterranean countries eat about 40 percent of their daily calories in the form of fat, they have a much lower rate of breast cancer than women in the United States. While these women eat more fat than American women, there is one important difference: They are more likely to use olive oil and, unlike American women, rarely use butter or margarine. In fact, according to one study from Greece, women who consume olive oil at more than one meal a day are much less likely to develop breast cancer than women who use less olive oil.

Fiber Many studies have shown a strong relationship between a diet high in fiber with lower rates of many different kinds of cancers, including breast cancer. The reason why fiber may protect against breast cancer is not fully understood, and there could be several explanations. Foods that are high in fiber, such as fruits and vegetables, are also rich in vitamins, minerals, and phytochemical compounds that may prove to be strong cancer protectors. In fact, researchers at the National Cancer Institute are investigating the cancer-fighting potential of a whole range of fruits and vegetables, and their findings may prove that food is potent medicine. Fiber may also help to maintain normal hormone levels, which could also help to protect against cancer. In a study conducted by the American Health Foundation, postmenopausal women ate 30 grams of wheat bran daily. After two months,

37

these women showed a marked reduction in blood levels of estradiol and estrone, two potent estrogens that are thought to stimulate the growth of breast tumors. A high-fiber diet may also help boost the body's immune system. A study from San Antonio's Cancer Research Center showed improved immune function in women on high-fiber, low-fat diets who have been treated for breast cancer. While the study only involved eight women, the findings are intriguing.

Restrict alcohol A high-alcohol intake has been associated with an increased incidence of breast cancer, as well as other types of cancers. One study showed that women who drink about an ounce of pure alcohol daily (about the amount in two average-size drinks) had higher blood and urine levels of potent forms of estrogen. This is of great concern since this particular type of estrogen has been shown to stimulate the growth of breast tumors.

Beta-carotene At least one study performed at the Department of Social and Preventive Medicine at the State University of New York at Buffalo compared the diets of over four hundred breast cancer patients with those of women who were cancer-free. The researchers found that the women who were cancer-free had a significantly higher intake of foods that were rich in beta-carotene, such as broccoli, apricots, carrots, and pumpkin. Although I don't think we should read too much into this one study, these are healthy foods that we should be eating anyway, and they may also protect against heart disease and other forms of cancer.

Soy foods Asians not only eat less fat than Westerners but they also eat vast quantities of foods derived from the soybean, notably tofu or bean curd. Compounds found in soy foods have been shown to block the growth of cancerous cells in test tube studies. In addition, soy foods contain isoflavones, compounds that are converted in the body to a weak form of estrogen called ekuol. Ekuol appears to bind to estrogen receptor sites on cells, preventing attachment of the more potent forms of estrogen that can cause tumors to grow.

General guidelines Although the data are unclear, I still believe that it makes good sense to restrict your intake of fat—especially saturated fat, which is found in dairy and meat, and transfatty acid, which is found in margarine—to 30 percent of daily calories. Even if reducing fat intake does not prevent breast cancer, there is excellent evidence that it will reduce the risk of cardiovascular disease, which is the number-one killer of American women, and will also protect against colon cancer.

Adding fresh fruits and vegetables to your diet is another way to reduce fat (most fruits and vegetables are very low in fat) and add fiber and other important substances found in these foods which may help protect against cancer.

Q. I am forty years old and very confused about mammograms. I have heard conflicting reports on the news as to whether women my age should have mammograms, and when I asked my doctors what they thought, I got different answers. My internist said that it might be advisable to have a mammogram now as a baseline, and then to follow up every few years or so with another. My gynecologist, however, said that she is still recommending that her patients over forty have an annual mammogram. Who should I listen to?

A. If you are confused about when to get a mammogram, you are not alone. In recent years, there has been a great deal of controversy over the age at which women should begin getting annual mammograms. Everyone agrees on one point: All women over fifty should have a mammogram each year. Whether women in their forties (or even earlier) should have annual mammograms or mammograms at all is a subject hotly debated by the medical community.

One problem with mammograms in women forty and under is that the breast tissue is often dense, which makes an accurate picture difficult to produce. Another problem is that there is conflicting evidence as to whether mammograms actually save lives.

Controversy over mammograms began in 1992 when a Canadian study reported finding more advanced cancers in women in their forties who had annual mammograms than in women who did not. The way in which the study was reported by the press erroneously suggested that mammograms were at best worthless and at worst responsible for promoting cancer in younger women. After careful review, most experts believed the study was poorly performed and, therefore, not valid. Nevertheless, the National Cancer Institute (NCI) withdrew its recommendations that women under fifty have routine mammograms on the grounds that it did not appear to prolong life (it did so over the objections of its own national advisory panel): Major medical groups, including the American Medical Association, also objected to the NCI's new guidelines. Although the NCI guidelines could not prevent women under fifty from getting mammograms, it did give insurance companies and HMOs a rationale for not offering to reimburse women in this age group for the test. In January 1995, another study, this one published in the *Journal of the American Medical Association*, found that mammograms offered little benefit in terms of survival rates in women under fifty.

The mammogram story is far from over: For every study that has shown mammograms to be worthless in women under fifty, there is another that shows them to be invaluable. In fact, according to the NCI, deaths from breast cancer are down 8 percent in white women in their forties since 1990, which is believed to be due primarily to mammograms. Two other major studies involving a total of 165,000 women have found improved survival rates for women between forty and forty-nine who had regularly scheduled mammograms. Perhaps what is even more important is that several studies have confirmed that mammograms are detecting breast cancer in women of all ages at much earlier stages, when the chances for survival or even a cure are at their best. According to Dr. Cody of Memorial Sloan-Kettering in New York, twenty years ago, before routine mammography, between 1 and 2 percent of all breast cancers were diagnosed in situ—that is, before it has spread beyond the breast—and the cure rate was close to 100 percent. Today, 20 percent of all breast cancers are diagnosed in situ, which has dramatically improved the prognosis for thousands of women. Early detection is of particular importance to young women, because premenopausal breast tumors tend to be aggressive and fast-growing. In weighing the results of all of these studies, I firmly believe that mammography is not only useful but essential for women in their forties. Here is the advice I give my patients:

- For high-risk women: If you have a mother, aunt, or sister who died of breast cancer before age forty, you should start having annual mammograms early, possibly in your twenties, definitely by age thirty-five. In addition to the annual mammogram, these women should have a physician (preferably a breast specialist) physically examine their breasts at least twice a year.
- For average-risk women: If you are not at any particular risk of getting breast cancer, you should have a baseline mammogram between the ages of thirty-five and forty. After age forty, I recommend that patients have mammograms at least every two years. By age fifty, all women should have annual mammograms. At any age, a woman should have an annual checkup in which a physician performs a physical examination of her breasts.

Q. *My doctor found a suspicious-looking spot on a mammogram and insisted that I have it biopsied. It turned out to be nothing more than a calcium deposit, but now I'm wondering why I had to go through all that discomfort and anxiety for nothing. Isn't there a way to diagnose breast cancer without having to resort to surgery?*

A. Given the fact that 90 percent of all breast lumps are benign, many patients who have undergone biopsies only to discover that there is nothing wrong often ask if the procedure was even necessary. Unfortunately, in many cases, biopsy is the only way to distinguish between a benign lump and one that is malignant. The good news is there are a few new procedures being tested that may eliminate the need to biopsy breast tissue in some cases. In one procedure, called scintimammography, a low-dose radioactive material called a tracer is injected into a woman's arm and travels throughout the bloodstream. The tracer illuminates breast cancers when photographed with a special camera. Early results look promising; in preliminary studies in small numbers (about 147 patients), the use of tracers seems to improve the ability of a mammogram to discern cancer from a benign lump. If this proves true in larger groups of patients, it might help avoid the need for painful, expensive, and possibly disfiguring biopsies. This can save the patient both wear and tear and money. Biopsies cost between $1,500 and $3,000. Scintimammography costs about $600 and gives off the same radiation as a cross-country airplane trip.

Another new technique involves putting sensors on the breast to detect abnormal electrical signals (much like, in principle, an electrocardiogram, which is used to assess the electrical state of the heart). A computer can then analyze areas of abnormal activity. A recent study from San Antonio correctly identified 178 of 182 biopsy-proven cancers and, equally important, said 181 of 210 benign lesions were, in fact, benign. More clinical experience with the testing is needed, though, before this technique can be used on patients.

Q. *I had my first mammogram at age thirty-eight. That was five years ago. It was so painful that I have been avoiding having another. Is there anything I can do to relieve the pain?*

A. Because we want to encourage women to get mammograms, most physicians do not talk about how mammograms can sometimes hurt. We use words like "discomfort" or "pressure" to describe what many women like yourself find to be uncomfortable and even painful. I think it is important for patients to be prepared so that they are not shocked by the experience. Yes, when the breasts are pressed between the plates, there may be some pain. The good news is, the pain is fleeting and lasts for no more than a few seconds at most.

There are always ways to reduce the pain. I advise women not to schedule mammograms at the time of their monthly cycle when their breasts are most tender, usually right before their periods. In addition, taking an Advil or two about an hour before the mammogram can significantly help relieve any pain or discomfort.

Q. *My mother died of breast cancer when she was fifty. I recently read about the discovery of a gene for breast cancer. Should I be tested? If I have inherited the gene from my mother, does it mean that I will definitely get breast cancer?*

A. Before I answer your question, let me reassure you that having a mother or a close relative who died of breast cancer does not automatically mean that you will also get breast cancer. Although the fact that your mother died of breast cancer does somewhat increase your risk, keep in mind that only 5-10 percent of all cases of breast cancer are believed to be due to an inherited genetic flaw. The overwhelming number of cases of breast cancer are due to other factors, many of which have not yet been identified.

In recent years, scientists have located two genes—BRCA1 and BRCA2—that are believed to predispose a woman to breast cancer, and other forms of cancer as well. A gene is a piece of genetic material that is located on the chromosomes that parents pass on to their young at conception. If a gene is defective, it could cause serious problems. In the case of BRCA1 and BRCA2, defects in these genes could possibly hamper the body's natural ability to weed out cancer cells. Women who inherit the BRCA1 gene stand an 85 percent chance of getting breast cancer by age seventy and a 40 percent chance of developing ovarian cancer; women who inherit the BRCA2 gene have a slightly higher than normal risk of getting breast cancer. Inheriting either BRCA gene increases the likelihood of colon cancer.

As of yet, we do not recommend widespread testing for either BRCA gene. Because these genes are capable of so many mutations—that is, they can easily change their structure, making them difficult to identify—screening is very difficult. Instead, I believe that women who are at high risk for breast cancer due to a strong family history should be scrupulous about getting annual mammograms. It is imperative that these women see breast specialists often—perhaps as often as every six months for a professional manual exam of their breasts.

Q. *I recently read that women who worked in jobs that increased their exposure to electromagnetic fields were more likely to develop breast cancer. A power line runs near my house; does this automatically increase my risk of breast cancer? Is it safe to use electrical appliances such as hair dryers or electric blankets?*

A. As the risk of developing breast cancer continues to rise, women are desperately looking for a culprit, particularly one that can be controlled. At the moment, electromagnetic fields (EMFs) are being blamed for the rise in breast cancer, and this has generated a great deal of controversy within the medical community. Although some scientists believe there is a direct link between exposure to EMFs and breast cancer, many others feel that there is a great deal more fear than actual fact.

Electromagnetic fields are invisible forces emitted by electricity. Anything that generates or runs on electricity—from power lines to computer screens to virtually every household appliance, radiates some level of EMFs. Concern over EMFs began several decades ago when studies suggested that there may be an increase in cancer among children who live near power lines. Follow-up studies have been inconclusive. One highly publicized study conducted by the University of North Carolina studied U.S. death records from 1985 to 1989. The researchers found that women who worked in electrical occupations had a 38 percent greater risk of developing breast cancer than women who did not work in these occupations. What was puzzling about this study, however, was that women who were in jobs that exposed them to the highest amount of EMFs actually had lower rates of breast cancer than women in white-collar, supervisory jobs who were not exposed to high levels of EMFs. One of the problems with this study was that it did not include interviews with the women themselves, who were already dead, but relied on second-hand information to determine if the women had described their occupations accurately. As a result, many scientists felt that this study had been poorly done, and dismissed the results. The National Cancer Institute is investigating the entire subject of EMFs and cancer risk, but it will be several years before any of its studies are completed.

People who believe that EMFs may increase the risk of cancer cite studies that show that exposure to electromagnetic fields can interfere with the brain's production of the key hormone melatonin. Several studies have documented that melatonin can inhibit the growth of breast cancer cells in laboratory tests, which suggests that it may play a similar role in the body. If melatonin does protect against cancer, then perhaps exposure to EMFs may indeed increase the risk of developing cancer. This is, however, all highly speculative and has never been proven in any clinical studies.

Before you panic and put your home up for sale, keep in mind that many scientists feel that this entire issue has been overblown. Recently, the American Physical Society, which include some of the nation's top physicists, did an intensive review of more than a thousand articles on EMFs and cancer risk. Based on this review, the group concluded that fears over EMFs were completely groundless.

As far as using appliances such as hair dryers or electric blankets, there is simply no evidence to suggest that these appliances are unsafe. For example, one recent study followed 380 women between the ages of forty-one and eighty-five who used electric blankets over a ten-year period. Researchers did not find a significantly increased risk of breast cancer.

In sum, there is little concrete evidence to link EMF exposure to breast cancer. At this point, it seems unnecessary to worry about unproven risks; your best rotection against breast cancer is to focus on the known risk factors: do not smoke, avoid excessive alcohol consumption, maintain normal body weight, and reduce your intake of dietary fat.

Q. *When I was a little girl, my parents used to have our lawn sprayed with DDT every summer. Now I hear that DDT may cause breast cancer. Since I have been exposed to this pesticide, am I now at greater risk of getting breast cancer?*

A. We do not know for sure. DDT (dichloro-diphenyl-trichloro-ethane) was banned in 1972 because it was shown to induce cancers, including breast tumors, in laboratory animals. Some studies have shown higher than normal rates of breast cancer among women who have elevated levels of DDT in their breast tissue either from working in the chemical industry or from having been exposed to the pesticide in other ways. A major study, however, conducted by the Kaiser Foundation Research Institute in Oakland, California, did not find that breast cancer patients had higher blood levels of DDE—a residual chemical of DDT that is stored in body fat and would have indicated early exposure than women who did not develop cancer.

Although there are no concrete answers as to whether DDT exposure increases the risk of breast cancer, scientists are beginning to shed light on the way this pesticide may behave in the body, which may one day help to solve the cancer question. When DDT is broken down in the body, it is converted into an even more potent chemical that mimics the action of hormones such as estrogen. Here's how it may work: When natural estrogen circulates throughout the body, it links onto certain cells via special structures called estrogen receptors. Once the estrogen binds with the receptor, it can trigger various activities, including cell growth. Some particularly strong forms of estrogen are believed to stimulate the growth of tumors. As DDT circulates throughout the body, some researchers believe that it may fool the estrogen receptors into believing that it is the real thing, enabling it to link up with the estrogen receptor and thus begin the chain of events that will eventually lead to the growth of breast tumors.

Other commonly used chemicals, including petroleum by-products and polychlorinated biphenyls (PCBs) are believed to have smilar estrogenic action in the body, and have also been investigated as potential causes of breast cancer.

Given the contradictory studies, I would not be too worried about the fact that you were exposed to DDT early in life. I would, however, be scrupulous about getting annual mammograms and examining my breasts monthly, as any woman should be.

Breast discharge

Q. *Although it has been years since I have nursed a baby, when I was examining my breasts recently I noticed that one nipple produced a small amount of milk. What could be causing this? Is it cause for concern?*

A. What you are describing is galactorrhea, a condition in which a woman produces milk although she is not breast feeding. Galactorrhea can be caused by several things, including a hormonal imbalance or a benign tumor of the pituitary. In addition, some women may find that their nipples secrete a milky discharge when they are sexually aroused or under stress. In some cases, drugs—including birth control pills, marijuana, and antidepressants—may be throwing the hormone balance out of whack. Usually this condition is not serious. As a rule, however, women should check with their doctors if they detect any discharge from their nipples, including a milky fluid, blood, or pus.

Implants

Q. *I have silicon breast implants and I'm worried that the implants will mask any lumps or tumors that could be cancerous. Is this a problem? Am I at greater risk of getting breast cancer?*

A. Both patients and doctors worry that breast implants will make it more difficult to perform both mammography and physical examinations. These fears, however, may not be based on fact. According to Dr. Cody at Memorial Sloan-Kettering, breast implants should not prevent a doctor from doing a thorough manual examination of the breast. For one thing, the typical patient with breast implants usually has a relatively small amount of breast tissue, which can make it easier to detect any lumps than in a woman with bigger breasts. For another, when the implant is inserted, the breast tissue is stretched over the surface of the implant, which may actually make it easier to see and feel lumps than without the implant. Nor does Dr. Cody believe that implants increase the risk of breast cancer, or interfere in any way with obtaining an accurate diagnosis. In fact, in his experience, when women with implants do develop cancer, it is usually diagnosed very early, probably due to the fact that their breasts are easy to examine. His observations are confirmed by a major Canadian study of women with breast implants that concluded, "the incidence of breast cancer among the women who had breast augmentation could not be said to be either significantly higher or lower than that among the general population."

On the question of whether or not implants interfere with mammography, I checked with New York plastic surgeon Alan M. Engler, who has many patients with breast implants. Dr. Engler said that in some cases an implant may restrict the ability of a mammogram to detect cancer, but this problem is not insurmountable. He advises his patients to alert the mammographer about the implants. A skilled mammographer should be able to manipulate the breast and take extra views so that the mammogram is nearly as accurate as one without implants.

Q. *I have had silicone breast implants for ten years. Although I have had no problems with them, I have heard things about implants that worry me. Are they dangerous? Should I have them removed?*

A. Since they were first offered in 1963, more than a million American women have received silicone gel-filled breast implants either to enlarge or reshape their breasts. Many women with breast cancer have also opted for silicone implants following reconstructive surgery after mastectomy.

Starting in the 1980s, there have been widely publicized reports of problems associated with silicone gel implants, including hardening of the breasts, ruptured implants causing pain and inflammation, and even cases of scleroderma, an arthritis-like disease that can cause pain and swelling in the joints. There have also been claims that silicone breast implants have increased the risk of developing serious autoimmune diseases such as systemic lupus erythematosus (SLE) and rheumatoid arthritis. There have been numerous lawsuits against the manufacturers of silicone gel implants; and in 1993, a federal judge set aside $4.25 billion to compensate the more than 400,000 women who have made claims asserting that their silicone gel implants made them ill. The money has yet to be divided up. Because of the questions raised about implants, in 1992 the Food and Drug Administration restricted the use of silicone gel breast implants in all cases except for reconstructive surgery after mastectomy. There is one kind of breast implant that is still available in the United States: a silicone-covered implant that is filled with a saline solution (salt and water) instead of silicone gel. Saline implants are considered safer because if they rupture, unlike silicone gel, the saline solution is easily absorbed by the body with no apparent ill effects. Silicone gel implants, however, are still available in Canada and Europe with no restrictions.

There is no doubt that some women with silicone gel implants did suffer problems that resulted in pain and disfigurement, and that if the implant ruptured, some women did have problems related to the silicone gel. What is in doubt, however, is the link between silicone gel implants and autoimmune disease. In fact, several well-done, serious studies did not find any association between breast implants and an increased risk of autoimmune diseases, and many rheumatologists are dubious that such a link actually exists.

More studies are being done to determine if silicone gel implants are indeed dangerous. At this point, I would not advise a patient to have her implants removed unless she is experiencing any untoward symptoms, or is unduly nervous about the possibility that she may develop a problem.

Q. *I would like my breasts to be larger, but I don't want to get breast implants. Are there any other options?*

A. There is no way short of breast enhancement surgery to actually increase the size of your breasts, but there are ways to make them appear to be larger.

Very often, better muscular support for your breasts will make them seem bigger. To achieve better support for your breasts, you need to do exercises that will strengthen your pectoral muscles, the muscles that connect the wails of the chest to the bones of the upper arms and shoulders. If you go to a gym or health club, ask the trainer what machines can help you firm and strengthen the muscles of your chest and back. Women often have poor upper-body strength and look flabby and poorly defined from the waist up. A good exercise program will improve the shape and contours of your breasts and back. There are also two exercises that you can do at home that are particularly effective:

Rubberband stretch Either sitting or standing, hold a thick rubberband (available at sports centers) between your fists at chest level. Start at a relaxed position. Stretch as far as you can. Hold for a count of 4 and then release slowly. Repeat exercise 10 times. Do two more sets of 12.

Prayer positioning Place your palms together and hold them chest high in a praying position. Press your palms together until you feel the muscles of your chest contract. Hold the pressure for a count of 4 and then slowly release. Repeat exercise 10 times. Do two more sets of 10.

Since the controversy over surgical breast implants, many new breast enhancement products have come on the market that can be worn under clothes, including inserts made of silicone gel that can be placed inside a bra or bathing suit. Unlike the typical padded bras of the past, silicone bra inserts mold to your shape and do not create an unnaturally stiff or cone-shaped appearance. These products are available through catalogues, at better lingerie stores, or at stores that specialize in bras for women who have had mastectomies. The only downside is that some of these breast enhancing products are expensive (they can cost more than $100), but considering the pain and cost of surgery, in my opinion, they are a true bargain.

Caffeine

Q. *I need a cup or two of coffee in the morning to get me going. My daughter, who follows a strict macrobiotic diet, has been nagging me about my coffee drinking. She contends that caffeine (I only drink caffeinated coffee) is an addictive drug that can cause all kinds of health problems. I have already stopped smoking and am on a strict low-fat diet. Do I really have to give up coffee?*

A. Before I answer your question, let me tell you about an experience I recently had. Unbeknownst to me, my secretary decided that caffeine was unhealthy and began bringing me decaffeinated coffee in the morning. For days, I suffered from terrible headaches that nothing seemed to help. Seeing how miserable I was, my assistant finally confessed to what she had done and brought me a cup of *real* coffee. Miraculously, my headaches disappeared and I felt like my energetic self again.

I know from firsthand experience that caffeine is addicting. Although we don't tend to think of it as such, caffeine is a drug—in fact, it is the most widely used drug in the world. Caffeine is found in foods, including chocolate, and beverages other than coffee, including tea and cola drinks. It is estimated that about 80 percent of the U.S. population ingests caffeine in some

48

form during the day. Once you begin using caffeine, it is hard to quit. Even moderate caffeine users who abstain from caffeine for even one day will experience withdrawal, including headache, fatigue, and flulike symptoms. This does not mean, however, that caffeine or coffee is dangerous. Even though caffeine is addictive, the amount that is normally found in one or two cups of coffee or tea appears to be harmless. For some, it may even be beneficial. For example, caffeine can improve mental alertness, combat fatigue, and even increase metabolism, which can help burn fat. Caffeine is also an excellent treatment for migraine headache since it dilates the blood vessels in the brain, thus reducing pain. The excessive use of caffeine is an entirely different issue. Too much caffeine—more than four or five cups daily—can cause nervousness, insomnia, aggravate high blood pressure, and even trigger heart palpitations in some people. Although caffeine is a stimulant, a high dose of caffeine over time can have just the opposite effect, especially if consumed with a sugary treat such as a doughnut. Both caffeine and sugar can cause a sudden surge in insulin, a hormone produced by the pancreas, which will put the body into overdrive, resulting in a mid-morning slump.

There have been many studies on the health effects of coffee and some have been extremely negative. For example, in 1981, a highly publicized study linked coffee drinking—with or without caffeine—to a substantially increased risk of pancreatic cancer. Another study linked coffee drinking to bladder cancer. And since there have been anecdotal reports linking caffeine to fibrocystic breast disease, some researchers speculated that it may also increase the risk of breast cancer. More recent studies, however, have not found any relationship between coffee and cancer of any kind. In fact, on closer examination of some of these studies, researchers concluded that coffee was not the culprit, but that cigarette smoking was actually the cause of the increased cancer risk. Smokers drink twice as much coffee as nonsmokers, so although it appeared as if people who consumed the most coffee had the highest risk of cancer, in reality, the real risk was from their smoking.

Heavy caffeine users, however, do increase their risk of osteoporosis, a major threat for women. Women who drink caffeinated beverages lose more calcium in their urine than women who abstain from caffeine. In fact, according to the famous Nurses' Study (conducted by Harvard Medical School investigators who followed every conceivable aspect of the health and habits of over 100,000 nurses for several decades), women who consumed more than 817 milligrams of caffeine daily (roughly the amount in six to seven cups of coffee) were at three times the risk of suffering a hip fracture. There is some good news to this story, at least for moderate coffee drinkers: Drinking just one glass of milk daily can replace the calcium loss caused by two cups of coffee.

49

If you drink caffeinated coffee in moderation and are not showing any ill effects, there is no need to stop. I would recommend, however, that you drink a glass of low-fat milk or eat a yogurt daily to restore the lost calcium. I am not, however, giving caffeinated coffee even in small amounts a clean bill of health for everyone. Pregnant women in particular should be cautious about caffeine use. Some studies have linked caffeine to delayed conception, premature birth, and fetal-growth retardation, although others have not found any link. Even though we do not know for certain whether caffeine is harmful to the fetus, it is advisable for women to avoid it during pregnancy. If you have high blood pressure or a heart condition, it is also wise to reduce your intake of caffeine.

Cancer (General)

Q. *It seems to me that when I was growing up, cancer was a rare disease—you hardly ever heard about it. Today, however, it seems as if it's a virtual epidemic. Is cancer on the rise? If so, why?*

A. In the past two decades, there has been an increase in the incidence of cancer in the United States, but as I will discuss later, it is hardly indicative of an epidemic. There certainly has been more public discussion about cancer than ever before, which I believe has had a positive effect on alerting the public to this important health problem.

At one time, in the not too distant past, cancer was not considered a proper topic of conversation in polite society. The very word *cancer* elicited terror in the hearts of people who believed that the diagnosis was an automatic death sentence. Cancer patients and their family members often kept their disease a secret. The good news is, within the past two decades, we have made spectacular strides in the treatment of many different types of cancers. Cancer patients are living longer than ever before, and in fact, the death rates for many different forms of cancer are actually declining. As cancer becomes more treatable, cancer patients are becoming more open about their disease,

51

and many are even "going public" by organizing lobbying groups to elicit financial support for medical research.

Despite the good news, the bad news is that cancer is on the rise. According to the National Cancer Institute (NCI), the incidence of cancer in women rose by more than 12 percent in the years 1975-91. Part of the reason why cancer rates are on the rise is the fact that people are living longer, and the longer one lives, the greater the risk of getting some form of cancer. Another reason is that our detection systems are much improved: We are finding cancers more frequently and finding them earlier.

The rise in cancer among women is primarily due to an increase in particular forms of cancer, notably breast, lung, and melanoma. From 1975 to 1991, there was a 30.1 percent increase in the incidence of breast cancer and a stunning 65.3 percent increase in the incidence of lung cancer. (Interestingly, during this period, lung cancer rose by only 2.5 percent in men.) There has also been a dramatic increase in melanoma, a potentially lethal form of skin cancer, in both sexes.

Although certain types of cancers are more prevalent among women today, there are particular reasons for this reported increase. For example, the rise in breast cancer may not be reflective of an actual rise in the number of women with breast cancer but may be due in large part to better diagnostic techniques—specifically, mammography—that detect tumors in their earliest stages. Prior to mammography, tumors were detected only when they were large enough to be felt; therefore, many cases of breast cancer were never diagnosed at all or missed until the disease had significantly progressed. In addition, there are lifestyle changes that have occurred within the past two decades that have also contributed to the rise in breast cancer. For example, more and more women are delaying childbearing until their thirties and are having fewer children. Many researchers believe that pregnancy actually protects women against breast cancer because it decreases exposure to the kinds of hormonal surges that occur during regular monthly menstruation which may trigger the growth of tumors.

Despite the publicity about breast cancer and the growing concern among women about this disease, more women will actually die of lung cancer this year than of breast cancer (56,000 deaths from lung cancer versus 46,000 deaths from breast cancer). The increase in lung cancer is indisputably due to the rise in cigarette smoking among women since World War II. In fact, according to the American Cancer Society, about 85 percent of all cases of lung cancer in women is primarily due to cigarette smoking. Today, about 27 percent of all women smoke, and although that represents a decline of 6 percent since 1965, it is still very high, and is reflected in the rate of lung cancer. Smoking is particularly dangerous for women. For reasons that are not

52

entirely understood, women who smoke appear to be twice as likely to get lung cancer as men who smoke. What is even more alarming is the increase in smoking rates among white teenaged girls. It is important to note that smoking is not just bad for the lungs, it also increases the risk of developing other cancers, including colon, breast, and bladder cancer.

The increased incidence of melanoma (up 41 percent) is attributed to increased exposure to the sun as a result of the obsession with tanning and sunbathing that was prevalent in the 1970s and 1980s. Although people are more cautious today about sun exposure, the long-term effects of early exposure are just being felt in terms of increased rates of all types of skin cancers. Some experts also believe that the thinning of the ozone layer—the protective layer of gas above the earth that filters out ultraviolet rays—may be causing the increase in skin cancer.

If there is one ray of hope to the rising cancer rates in women, it is that many cancers are preventable by simply not smoking and limiting one's exposure to the sun. In addition, regular mammograms can detect breast cancer at its earliest stages, in which the prognosis is excellent for long-term survival.

Q. *I have a friend who was the picture of health—she looked and felt wonderful—until she was diagnosed with a rare form of cancer. Within weeks of the onset of her chemotherapy treatments she looked and felt terrible and even lost her hair. This seemed crazy to me: How can someone who is so healthy be so sick? Would she have been better off without the chemotherapy?*

A. The fact that a seemingly perfectly healthy person could be harboring a serious cancer, and the fact that the chemotherapy can often seem to be more deadly than the disease itself, is one of the hardest things to explain to patients, their families, and concerned friends. In its earliest stages, cancer is often a symptomless disease. Until the cancer eats into a tissue supplied with nerves, or is compromising a vital function such as the ability to breathe, you can feel fine and not even suspect that you are sick.

At times it may seem nonsensical to make a "well" patient sick by giving her chemotherapy, and you may wonder why doctors do not wait until the patient begins to show symptoms. Chemotherapy is, after all, a controlled way of administering poison. Ideally, the poison will target the cancerous cells and spare the healthy ones, but there can be some very serious side effects to chemotherapy, including damage to important bone marrow cells. In addition, chemotherapy often leaves patients exhausted and feeling sick. There are good reasons, however, for subjecting patients to this treatment in the earliest stages of their disease. If the cancer is diagnosed and treated early, it may be possible to eradicate

53

it with fewer chemotherapy treatments than would be needed after the cancer has spread, thus sparing the patient both the discomfort and potential threat of side effects. There is also a much greater chance of long-term survival.

Do not judge your friend's progress by how she looks a few weeks after chemotherapy. Give her some time. Within six months to a year, many cancer patients begin to regain their strength and are back to normal.

Chest Pain at Night

Q. *I frequently wake up with pain in my chest. It goes away in a few minutes and it's not very painful. I think it's only indigestion, but could it be my heart? Should I call my doctor?*

A. Chest pain at night could be caused by any of several problems, and although it is usually not serious and is just indigestion, it could also be life-threatening. Here are some of the possible causes of chest pain and advice on how to deal with them.

Heart If you wake up with severe chest pain call your doctor for advice, particularly if this is the first time this has happened to you. You could be having a heart attack or be suffering from angina pectoris, a condition caused by not enough blood flowing to the heart muscle, which could eventually lead to a heart attack. Other symptoms that often accompany angina or a heart attack are feeling breathless, heart palpitations, or profuse sweating. In many cases, your doctor will be able to sort out over the telephone, what is causing your pain by listening to the description of your symptoms. If she suspects a heart problem, she may want to meet you at her office or the nearest emergency room. If your doctor is not available, go to the nearest emergency room yourself. Even if it turns out to be a false alarm, and you are only suffering from indigestion, it is better to err on the side of caution than to miss the first signs of a heart attack. The earlier you have treatment for a heart attack, the better your chances of survival and complete recovery.

Exertion If you are awakened by mild pain that disappears quickly, it may very well be due to overexertion of your chest muscles. Try to remember any new or different activity that may have triggered the pain. Carrying unusually heavy bundles, playing tennis after a long period of inactivity, even vigorous sex can all cause muscle soreness after a few hours or even a day after exertion. Aspirin or ibuprofen should relieve muscle soreness.

Stomach An inflamed stomach lining, too much acid in the stomach, or even irritation of the tube that leads from the mouth to the stomach can all cause chest pain. If you wake up in pain and suspect that it is due to an angry stomach, try getting up out of bed and standing upright for a while. An antacid like Tums or Mylanta may also help.

Chronic Fatigue Syndrome

Q. For the past few months, no matter how much sleep I get, I feel exhausted. Could I have chronic fatigue syndrome? What are the symptoms and how can I find out if I have it?

A. One of the most difficult symptoms to diagnose is a complaint of unusual, persistent, and unrelieved exhaustion or fatigue. Fatigue is a common symptom of literally scores of different problems, from rheumatoid arthritis to thyroid deficiency to severe depression. And as you have noted, it could also be due to chronic fatigue syndrome, a disorder that is loosely defined as debilitating fatigue of more than six-month duration that is not due to any discernible medical condition. Since fatigue is such a general symptom, anyone who suffers from excessive fatigue should be seen by a doctor for a thorough workup.

When someone walks into my office with a complaint of fatigue, I first try to pinpoint a physical cause of the problem. For example, a simple blood test can check for anemia, underactive or overactive thyroid function, and low potassium levels. All of these conditions can cause extreme fatigue, which is easy to remedy with appropriate medication. I also talk with my patient and try to obtain pertinent information on lifestyle and sleep patterns. For example, alcohol abuse can cause excessive fatigue, among other

57

symptoms. In fact, for some people, a few drinks at night can profoundly disrupt normal sleep patterns, resulting in daytime exhaustion. Another possibility is that a patient may be suffering from a sleep disorder called sleep apnea, in which she stops breathing in her sleep, often waking herself up at night. If this happens throughout the night, it can also cause chronic fatigue. There is also a chance that there is a psychological cause to the overwhelming feelings of fatigue, such as depression or anxiety. To add to the confusion, very often, when someone is exhausted from a physical ailment, it can trigger depression. The risk here is that the doctor will pick up on the depression but not identify the underlying physical cause. That is why, when it comes to diagnosing the cause of fatigue, the greatest challenge for the doctor is to be able to separate out the physical and emotional factors. This not only takes skill and experience but often requires spending time with the patient, at the very least taking a detailed medical history. Only when I have ruled out every other possibility do I then consider a diagnosis of chronic fatigue syndrome. Unfortunately, there is no one diagnostic test for this problem; it must be diagnosed based on specific criteria. In order to receive a diagnosis of chronic fatigue syndrome, a patient must have experienced:

- persistent, unexplained chronic tiredness of new or definite onset (it cannot be a lifelong problem)
- fatigue that is not relieved by rest and, after exertion, the patient feels much worse for a time lasting more than twenty-four hours
- difficulty concentrating and remembering facts severe enough to impair or compromise previous levels of occupational, social, and personal activity
- tenderness in the lymph nodes in the neck and/or under the arms
- muscle pain and pain in the joints without swelling or redness
- headaches of a new type, pattern, or severity
- unrefreshing sleep

The cause of chronic fatigue syndrome has perplexed doctors for decades. The mystery, however, is slowly beginning to be unraveled. Prior to the onset of fatigue, many patients report a severe illness, such as an especially bad case of flu. This has led researchers to suspect that a virus such as Epstein-Barr or herpes may somehow be involved. Indeed, some patients with chronic fatigue syndrome do show high levels of antibodies to the Epstein-Barr and other viruses; on the other hand, many do not.

Some studies have linked extreme stress, such as a death in the family or divorce, as factors that may contribute to the onset of chronic fatigue syndrome. Although there is no concrete evidence that this is true, we do know that stress can have a profound effect on the immune system, our body's natural defense system against disease. If the immune system is weakened, it could leave the body vulnerable to infection.

A groundbreaking study that was published in the *Journal of the American Medical Association* appears to be a major breakthrough in revealing the cause of chronic fatigue syndrome, at least in many patients. The study, which included twenty-three patients with chronic fatigue syndrome, found that twenty-two of them had an abnormality in the way their bodies regulated blood pressure, which caused their hearts to slow down at precisely the times when it needed to speed up. For example, during periods of exertion, when you get up out of a chair, you need a stronger heartbeat to pump blood throughout the body. In individuals with chronic fatigue syndrome, however, the heartbeat did not speed up when it should, and actually slowed down. Oddly enough, this particular kind of low blood pressure cannot be diagnosed by the standard blood pressure test. Instead, the patient must be tilted at a 70-degree angle to the floor to simulate standing for a long period of time, the kind of exertion that can trigger the low blood pressure response. According to this study, during the tilt test, the patients with chronic fatigue syndrome and low blood pressure reported feeling lightheaded, faint, and nauseous and even felt lethargic and fatigued for days after the test. Researchers believe that if this low blood pressure response occurs often enough during the day, it could be the cause of the continual exhaustion.

Most of the patients in the study were successfully treated with medication to control blood pressure and an increased intake of salt and fluid. Out of the twenty-two patients who had low blood pressure, nine reported full recovery after treatment and seven said that their condition had improved.

One fact puzzling researchers is that there are many people with this type of low blood pressure who do not develop chronic fatigue syndrome. This has led researchers to speculate that a viral infection or some other illness must somehow trigger chronic fatigue syndrome in people with this kind of low blood pressure, and perhaps this blood pressure condition makes people susceptible to chronic fatigue syndrome. More studies are needed to determine if low blood pressure is truly the cause of chronic fatigue syndrome in many patients.

In the meantime, there are few effective treatments for chronic fatigue syndrome. Aspirin, acetaminophen, or nonsteroidal anti-inflammatory drugs can help relieve the headache and muscle pain. Antidepressants have also been helpful for many patients, and many others have found relief by practicing relaxation techniques such as yoga and deep breathing.

The one good thing about chronic fatigue syndrome is that the symptoms tend not to worsen over time, and there is no evidence of long-term physical deterioration. In fact, many patients do eventually recover.

Combat

Q. *Are women physically and emotionally strong enough for combat?*

A. Through the years, women have been told that they cannot participate in many occupations, ranging from law to medicine to engineering to construction work—because it allegedly went against the laws of nature. Today we know this is nonsense, and in fact, women are not only capable of performing the same tasks as men but often can do them as well or even better. Periodically, politicians who want to turn back the clock on women's rights— or who want to pander to men (or women) who may feel displaced by successful women—focus on the issue of limiting women's role in the military. It is an issue that is based on emotion rather than fact. People of either sex can be physically and psychologically strong enough for combat. Nothing about being female compromises building a strong body, having intelligence, courage, and the other emotional and mental resources that equip people to endure hardship.

Contraception

Q. *What is the best over-the-counter contraceptive?*

A. A latex condom used with spermicide containing nonoxynol-9 is the best form of contraception available without a doctor's prescription. If used vigilantly and correctly, the condom/spermicide combination provides excellent protection against pregnancy and sexually transmitted diseases. Natural skin condoms do not provide adequate protection against sexually transmitted diseases because they are too porous and should not be used for this purpose.

Q. *Does the female condom work as well as the male condom?*

A. Similar to the male condom, the female condom, which was approved by the Food and Drug Administration in 1992, is sold over-the-counter at drugstores. The female condom is a resilient polyurethane sheath that loosely fits over the opening of the cervix, covering the vaginal wall, creating a lined pathway for the penis. If correctly used, it is nearly as effective at preventing pregnancy as the male condom (there is a 12 percent failure rate for the male condom as compared to a 13 percent failure rate for the female condom).

The relatively high failure rate for both types of condoms is largely attributed to improper use, or in many cases, nonuse (in other words, the condom remains in the wrapper). Similar to the male condom, the female condom offers excellent protection against sexually transmitted diseases. One obvious advantage of the female condom over the male condom is that the former can be inserted several hours before intercourse; thus, there is no interruption during lovemaking. A negative: Some women find it too noisy to use, complaining that during thrusting the sheath moves back and forth, making an unpleasant sound.

In one important way the female condom is superior to the male condom: It helps women to take better care of themselves. Many women tell me that they have difficulty asking their partners to use condoms, and even if they do ask, their partners are sometimes reluctant to oblige. The female condom eliminates the need for that discussion, and empowers a woman to provide her own protection without the cooperation of her partner. I think the female condom is also an excellent choice for women who are taking birth control pills but who need extra protection against sexually transmitted diseases.

Birth control pills

Q. *After years of fussing with creams and diaphragms I am considering taking birth control pills. I have heard, however, that the Pill can increase the risk of cancer. Is this true? Is the Pill safe?*

A. It all depends on who is taking it. First introduced in the United States in the 1960s, birth control pills today are used by close to 11 million American women. After tubal ligation and vasectomy, the Pill is the most popular form of contraception. It has its appeal: There is no mess, no fuss, and it does the job. Few women who use the Pill consistently and correctly will have an unintended pregnancy (the failure rate is a mere .1 percent). Given the large number of women who use the Pill, its safety record is impressive. There is no widespread evidence that the Pill is dangerous for most women. This does not mean, however, that it is for everyone. There are some women who, due to their family medical history or a preexisting condition of their own, should not use the Pill. Other women may find that they experience uncomfortable side effects when on the Pill, such as headaches or excess bloating, and would do better using other methods of contraception. In any case, before a woman begins taking birth control pills, I strongly believe that she should be aware of the risks as well as the benefits. No woman should begin birth control pills without first being carefully examined by her physician to make sure there is nothing in her medical history that precludes her from using oral contraceptives. Any woman on the Pill should be closely monitored by her doctor. Women who smoke should use another means of contraception. (Research done on older forms of oral contraception that contained higher doses of estrogen than we use today when combined with smoking increased risk for coronary artery disease fortyfold. The same observations need to be made with the newer forms of OC's to decide whether women who use them and smoke are taking an unacceptable risk.)

Before I even discuss the pros and cons of the Pill, you need to know that the Pill does not offer protection against sexually transmitted diseases such as chlamydia and AIDS. Unless you are in a long-term relationship with a partner you know well and trust, you will still need to have your partner use a latex condom, or you will need to use a female condom to protect against disease.

How the Pill works Most birth control pills contain a combination of hormones—estrogen and progesterone—which in high enough doses, can inhibit ovulation, thus preventing the egg from developing normally in the ovaries. Without an egg, there can be no pregnancy. (Some women who cannot take estrogen may be given the so-called mini-pill, which is only synthetic progesterone.)

The cancer question Some studies have suggested that women who have used the pill for ten years or more are at somewhat greater risk of getting breast cancer than non-Pill users. Why? Both estrogen and progesterone can stimulate the growth of certain types of tumors—called hormone dependent tumors because they respond to hormonal stimulus. About two thirds of all breast tumors are hormone dependent. There is much debate in the medical community, however, over whether the Pill actually increases the risk of breast cancer, and many doctors simply do not believe it is true. When birth control pills were first offered, the doses of hormones were substantially higher than they are now. Many of the studies on the Pill were done on the high-dose pills; therefore, it is unlikely that these studies are applicable to the new, safer, low-dose pills. Because of the uncertainty, some doctors will not prescribe birth control pills to women with a strong family history of breast cancer. On the other hand, many oncologists believe that the Pill may actually protect against breast cancer by dampening the effects of the body's naturally produced hormones that may stimulate tumor growth. Only time—and more studies—will tell who is right.

What many women do not know is that birth control pills appear to offer strong protection against two cancers of the reproductive tract: ovarian cancer and endometrial cancer (cancer of the lining of the uterus). Out of the general population, 1 in 70 women will develop ovarian cancer in her lifetime.

If a woman has a strong genetic susceptibility to the disease—for example, if she has two or more first-degree relatives (mother, sister, or daughter) with ovarian cancer—her lifetime risk of developing ovarian cancer could be as high as 50 percent. According to a recent study, if high-risk women use birth control pills for at least ten years, their risk of developing ovarian cancer is actually lower than normal-risk women who have never used the Pill.

Heart disease Because women are so focused on cancer, they tend to forget that heart disease is actually the number-one killer of women. As a researcher in cardiology, I have some concerns about the potentially hazardous effects of the Pill on some women. About 5 percent of all women on the Pill will develop high blood pressure within a five-year period (as defined as any reading of 140/90 or above). High blood pressure can dramatically increase the risk of a heart attack or stroke. Although many of these studies linking high blood pressure to the Pill were done on the higher-dose pills, nevertheless, I am still concerned about the potential for trouble. Therefore, I would not recommend birth control pills to any woman with high blood pressure. If a woman is on the Pill, she should have her blood pressure checked at regular intervals by her physician.

The Pill's effect on cholesterol levels is also problematic. In some people, the progesterone component of the Pill may raise overall cholesterol levels, in particular, elevating levels of LDL ("bad cholesterol"), which increases the risk of heart disease. On the other hand, estrogen can lower LDL cholesterol and raise the levels of HDL ("good cholesterol"), which is beneficial. Estrogen, however, can also raise levels of triglycerides, another type of blood lipid that, if elevated (over 199 mg./dl.), can substantially increase a woman's risk of heart disease. Some studies have shown that some women on the Pill will experience a rise in bad cholesterol and triglycerides. Although many of these studies were done on the higher-dose pills, even one study using a commonly prescribed low-dose pill showed a mild increase in LDLs. Therefore, I feel that women with high cholesterol levels (anything over 220 mg./dl.) should not be given birth control pills. Once a woman is on the Pill, she should have her blood lipids measured every six months to make sure they are within the normal range.

The progesterone component of the Pill may also cause an increase in appetite, resulting in weight gain. Since being overweight is a major risk factor for heart disease, the Pill may not be an appropriate contraceptive for women who have a weight problem.

Finally, estrogen has been shown to promote blood clots, which can cause heart attack, stroke, and pulmonary embolisms (lung clots). (Since smokers are also more prone to develop blood clots, this is yet another reason why the

64

Pill and smoking do not mix.) I would not recommend any woman with a strong family history of blood clots or stroke to take the Pill.

Any woman on the Pill should be aware of the following warning signals. If you experience any of the following symptoms, call your doctor immediately:

- swelling or pain in the legs
- yellowing of skin or eyes
- pain in the abdomen
- shortness of breath
- severe headaches
- severe depression
- blurred or double vision

Q. *I have a friend who told me that she got pregnant while taking birth control pills because she did not know that the antibiotic prescribed by her doctor for a throat infection would reduce the effectiveness of the Pill. Could this be true?*

A. Yes. Many drugs can interact with the Pill and make it less effective, among them are some of the most commonly prescribed antibiotics like tetracycline or ampicillin. Anticonvulsant medication such as phenobarbital or primidone, tranquilizers such as Valium, and antifungal drugs like griseofulvin can also interfere. The bottom line is: If you are taking the Pill and your doctor prescribes any medication, be sure to remind her that you are on birth control pills. Do not assume that your doctor will remember. Be sure to ask specifically if a drug will alter the effectiveness of the Pill. If it does, you will need to use an additional form of contraception while you are taking the medication and perhaps for some time afterward.

Q. *I read in a vitamin guide that women who take the Pill need to take additional vitamins. I'm on the Pill: What vitamins should I be taking?*

A. Women on the Pill do need more of some vitamins and minerals than non-pill users. In particular, you need additional vitamin C, B6, B12, and folic acid. In addition to eating well, you should take a good multivitamin and mineral supplement daily.

Q. *My doctor took me off the Pill seven years ago, when I turned forty, because he said it was not safe for a woman my age to take it any longer. I have a close friend who is my age who is still taking the Pill. Recently, my periods have become very heavy and irregular (my body used to work like clockwork) and I have begun to experience some of the symptoms of menopause such as vaginal dryness and fatigue, but my friend on the Pill is experiencing none of these changes. In fact, she said that she is as regular as ever and has never felt better. Could the reason that she is doing so much better than me be that she is still on the Pill?*

A. At one time, doctors used to routinely take women off the Pill at around age thirty-five because the long-term effects of oral contraceptives were still unknown. Several recent studies have confirmed that the Pill—especially the new low-dose ones are safe for nonsmoking women throughout their forties. In fact, the FDA has approved the use of the Pill for women up to the age of fifty. Today, as many as 1.5 million women past the age of forty are on the pill.

There are several benefits to taking the Pill right up until menstruation ends. The Pill is an excellent contraceptive, and even though a woman is nearing menopause, it does not mean that she is not capable of getting pregnant. The reduction in menstrual cycles may give a false sense of security, but unless a couple is using contraception, there is always a risk of pregnancy. The Pill can also relieve much of the discomfort associated with the transition from the end of menstruation to menopause. As women approach menopause, they typically go through a period known as perimenopause in which they often have erratic periods characterized by either very heavy bleeding or breakthrough bleeding. Breakthrough bleeding is more than just an annoyance, it is a sign of a more serious problem and must be investigated—a process that can often lead to medical tests that are both anxiety-provoking and uncomfortable. Women on the Pill, however, are getting a steady dose of estrogen, which will keep their periods regular and spare them many of the other unpleasant symptoms of perimenopause and menopause. In many cases, women on the Pill will not even know when they become menopausal. Therefore, it may be necessary for these women to take a blood test, in which their hormone levels will be altered accordingly, to determine if they have reached menopause. (The Pill contains higher levels of estrogen and progesterone than hormone replacement therapy.)

If you are interested in going back on the Pill, talk to your doctor about whether you are a good candidate.

Q. *Is the "morning-after pill" safe? Does it work? Is there anything that you can do the morning after to protect yourself against sexually transmitted diseases?*

A. There are several regimens of hormones that can be used within a short period after sexual intercourse to prevent pregnancy. The "morning-after" pill that is most often used today is a higher than normal dose of the combination birth control pill Ovral. The usual protocol is two 50-mg. Ovral pills within seventy-two hours of unprotected intercourse, followed by two more 50-mg. pills twelve hours later. Although this method is not foolproof, the failure rate—that is, the rate of pregnancy—among women who follow this regimen is extremely low. Keep in mind, however, that the risk of actually conceiving after one unprotected intercourse mid-cycle is also fairly low (between 1 in 6 and 1 in 4 women). The FDA has not approved Ovral for this use and there have not been any studies on the long-term effects of this treatment.

I do not recommend that you try this regimen on your own. Heavy doses of hormones can throw your natural hormonal balance out of kilter, and it is advisable to discuss the potential effect of this treatment with your doctor before doing this by yourself. In addition to upsetting your own menstrual patterns, other side effects include extreme nausea, headaches, and dizziness.

The treatment of many sexually transmitted diseases is now simpler than it used to be: Often, a single dose of medication is all that is required. For example, gonococcal urethritis can be treated with one dose of an antibiotic like ciprofloxacin (400 mg. one time). A single oral one gram dose of azithromycin cures chlamydial urethritis and cervicitis. If you develop urinary tract symptoms after intercourse (burning, urgency) or have a vaginal discharge that seems unusual to you, see your doctor at your earliest opportunity for appropriate cultures and treatment. Some women develop urinary tract infections very frequently and these infections are related to sexual activity. If this is the case with you, your doctor may counsel you that one dose of an antibiotic medication the next day is in order. Be sure not to do this on your own, since the wrong medication or one taken for too short a time may well result in the development of organisms that are resistant to medication.

Death and Dying

Q. *What is the difference between being in a coma and being brain dead? When are you considered officially dead?*

A. A coma is a state of impaired consciousness that can vary in intensity. Doctors gauge the depth of coma by noting whether the patient responds to outside stimuli and whether automatic processes like breathing or body temperature control are impaired. If the areas of the brain that control automatic functions continue to operate, breathing and heartbeat continue, although the patient may not hear or be able to react to outside stimuli.

The causes of coma vary: some are due to structural damage after a head injury, others are due to poisoning or metabolic imbalances caused by disease. The electroencephalogram (EEG), which uses electrodes attached to the scalp to record the electrical activity of the brain, is very useful in helping doctors decide what is causing the depressed state of consciousness.

When a patient is brain dead, there is no electrical activity on the EEG and there are no brain stem reflexes for at least twelve hours. A brain-dead patient in whom no electrical activity can be demonstrated after twenty-four hours is officially dead, although automatic functions like breathing can be maintained indefinitely by external machines.

Q. *If had a terminal illness and was in a great deal of pain, would my doctor help me to end my life quickly and painlessly?*

A. This is one of the most controversial issues in medicine today. The Hippocratic oath, which states, "First, do no harm," forbids a physician's doing anything intentional to end the patient's life, like injecting a large bolus of air into a vein. On the other hand, the doctor's responsibility not to prolong a doomed patient's life with temporary measures like a respirator, when there is no real advantage in providing the patient with a few more days of existence, is a very serious one. Adequately treating pain in the dying patient is an important responsibility of the physician. Any reasonable physician would give you enough medication to eliminate pain, even if an unwanted or unwarranted side effect was to depress breathing.

Q. *After watching my aunt die a slow and painful death from cancer, I decided that if I had a terminal illness I would not want to be kept alive at any cost. What do I need to do to ensure that this will not happen to me?*

A. I recommend that you give your physician a document called a living will in which you clearly state the precise extent of what you want in terms of intervention in the event of a fatal illness. The decision about when "enough is enough" should be made well in advance wherever possible while you are well, or at least while you are conscious and rational. Your doctor must know what you mean when you say you wish to die as comfortably as possible.

There are several stages to that discussion. Once it is established that the patient cannot recover meaningful function after an event like a stroke or an illness like widespread cancer, several points are important. Do you want any infection treated with antibiotics? A patient with metastatic cancer, for example, may well get a pneumonia that threatens her life. She may, if the pneumonia is treated with antibiotics, choose to have such a treatment so that she can have more months of life. On the other hand, if her death is anticipated within a very short time, treating the pneumonia may unnecessarily prolong her suffering. Death from pneumonia or death as a result of blood loss may be much more comfortable than other possible modes of exit.

The same principles are true of fluid replacement by vein, artificial feeding through a tube placed inside a blood vessel or into the stomach, attaching a patient to a respirator or transfusing a patient with blood or blood products. All of these decision points should be discussed ahead of time and recorded in a "living will." Copies of a suggested living will can be gotten from your local medical society.

You may want to refuse all supportive measures in the belief that it will speed things along, but I would advise a clause that stipulates that you do want all measures to increase your comfort level. This includes IV fluids to prevent dehydration (a very uncomfortable form of death) and adequate medication for pain.

Many doctors will provide an outline of a living will for you to follow. I would also recommend that you discuss your concerns with your doctor so that she can help you decide what to include in your living will.

I also recommend that you talk to your lawyer about designating a close friend or relative as your health care proxy. This would empower him or her to make decisions about what is acceptable treatment in the event that a specific situation is not covered in your living will.

The *Journal of the American Medical Association* reported a recent important and well-planned survey of patients from five medical centers around the country about how well patient's dying wishes were observed by their doctors. Half of terminally ill patients lived for eight days or more in what the authors called "undesirable states": they were in intensive care units, comatose, or on respirators. Half of all the dying patients were in considerable pain and discomfort. Discussions about the decisions the doctor and patients had to make were often much too delayed to make them useful: Nearly half of all "do not resuscitate" orders were written within forty-eight hours of the patient's death! Often doctors are pressured, particularly within hospital settings, to "do everything" for a patient; I have seen doctors give a transfusion or write an order for an antibiotic because of pressure from the nursing staff rather than because the intervention was in the best interest of the patient. If you have an incurable illness it is very helpful to talk with your doctor and family about not going to the hospital at all when your life is coming to an end. Your family should be an important part of the contract you sign with your doctor: They and you should try to agree ahead of time about each of the decisions that have to be made.

Diet

Q. *I have tried many different diets and have not been able to maintain the weight loss for more than a few months. A friend of mine told me that if I limit the number of fat grams, I can eat everything I want and not gain weight. Is this true? What do you think is the best way to lose weight?*

A. Your friend is absolutely wrong. In recent years, there has been an explosion in weight loss programs that are based on the premise that all it takes to keep off excess pounds is to limit your daily intake of fat grams. In other words, you can eat all the food you want as long as you do not exceed a designated number of fat grams. There is some rationale to this approach. Compared to other types of foods—protein and carbohydrates—fat is more fattening. One gram of fat weighs in at 9 calories, whereas one gram of carbohydrates and protein weighs in at 4 calories. Theoretically, you can eat more protein and carbohydrate than if you are loading up on the same amount of fat. Nevertheless, a calorie is a calorie is a calorie, and no matter how you try to bend the rules, the laws of thermodynamics still prevail. If you take in more calories than you burn—in any form—you will gain weight. There is no easy way around this equation.

It is interesting to note that since the growing popularity of diets based on counting fat grams, there has been a proliferation of no-fat and low-fat prod-

71

ucts on the market. Many of these products are laden with sugar and are actually quite high in calories. It is also interesting to note that despite the obsession with dieting, within the past decade Americans have actually put on weight. American adults, on average, weigh ten pounds more than they did a decade ago, according to a recent study by the National Center for Health Statistics. In fact, nearly one third of all adults are obese—weighing 20 percent or more above their desired body weight. Many experts believe that this national weight gain may in large part be due to the mistaken belief that a reduction in fat will automatically equal a reduction in weight.

Since there is so much confusion and misinformation on diet, I believe that the best way to lose weight and to keep it off is to work with a qualified nutritionist who will tailor a weight-loss program for you. Make sure your doctor monitors your serum fats as you diet: A woman's "good cholesterol" (HDL or high-density lipoproteins) level will drop along with the drop in total cholesterol and low-density lipoprotein (LDL, "bad cholesterol," which helps plug up arteries with plaques of fatty material). Levels of HDL above 45 are important for women; this "good cholesterol" helps keep blood vessels open and actually prevents plaque formation.

Q. *Can eating a lot of sugar make you diabetic?*

A. Yes, a diet high in sugar can increase the risk of developing one type of diabetes in susceptible people. There are two forms of diabetes: juvenile diabetes, also known as Type I or insulin-dependent diabetes, and adult-onset diabetes, also known as Type II, or non-insulin-dependent diabetes.

Juvenile diabetes occurs when the islet cells of the pancreas, which produce insulin, are destroyed by an autoimmune reaction. Insulin is critical for the breakdown of sugars and starches. As its name implies, juvenile diabetes most often strikes before age forty, often during childhood, and is treated with daily injections of insulin. People with juvenile diabetes must carefully monitor their intake of sugar and carbohydrates, which the body easily breaks down into sugar. This kind of diabetes cannot be precipitated by eating a lot of sugar.

Excess sugar intake can help cause or worsen the second, and the more common, type of diabetes—adult-onset diabetes. People with this type of diabetes not only have impaired insulin secretion but also tissue that is resistant to insulin's action. In a vicious circle, the high levels of sugar in the blood that result can produce further impairment of insulin secretion and tissue sensitivity to the hormone.

About 1 in 4 Americans has a genetic tendency to develop adult-onset diabetes, and it is twice as common in women as in men. A diet high in sugar can trigger this type of diabetes because it is constantly challenging the pancreas to produce insulin, and since tissue utilization of the insulin is defective, the hormone does not control the excess sugar.

Diabetes is a very serious risk factor for coronary artery disease, particularly in women, and removes any protection a woman has because she is still menstruating. Diabetes, whether juvenile or adult onset, carries with it not only the risk of heart attack but of stroke, kidney disease, blindness, and severe circulatory problems.

A recent study published in the *American Journal of Clinical Nutrition* investigated whether a high dietary sugar intake in the form of fructose—a sweetener that is widely used in prepared foods such as baked goods—can raise cholesterol, thus increasing the risk of heart disease. The study concluded that a high-fructose diet can not only raise cholesterol levels but can increase LDL ("bad cholesterol"), and triglycerides, which, if elevated, can increase the risk of heart disease in women. This study is particularly significant because many people consume high quantities of fructose in processed and prepared foods and are completely unaware of it. Limiting the amount of processed foods you eat is one way to avoid excess fructose.

Sugar is not the only culprit; there is evidence that a high-fat diet can also promote insulin resistance. Obesity, particularly if fat is concentrated around the abdomen ("central" obesity) is another culprit, which is why weight loss and exercise are so important in the control of diabetes. In fact, in some cases, a good program of weight loss and exercise can eliminate Type II diabetes altogether!

People who are overweight, or who have a family history of diabetes, should be careful about limiting their intake of sugar and fat, and should try to maintain a normal weight.

Digestive Disorders

Q. *I move my bowels every three days and I wonder if this is normal?*

A. Although the advertisements for commercial laxatives would have you think otherwise, there is a wide range of what is normal in terms of how frequently people move their bowels. For some people, moving their bowels once or twice a day is normal. Others move their bowels only once or twice a week. You should aim for elimination at least every third day; prolonged contact of waste matter with the colon increases your chances of colon cancer.

Constipation is usually temporary and caused by changes in lifestyle or diet: Frequent travelers, for example, often experience constipation because of irregular schedules, unfamiliar surroundings and foods, and time pressure. Chronic constipation can have a number of causes; your doctor can recommend a whole series of tests to decide on what the problem actually is. Thyroid malfunction, colonic inflammation, or tumor can all cause constipation. Some patients have impaired colonic motility; others have a weakness or malfunction of the pelvic muscles that help evacuate stool from the body. The remedies are as varied as the causes; laxatives are usually only a temporary solution. But biofeedback, pelvic muscle retraining, and even surgery can all help.

Your bowel movements should not be difficult or painful. If you have discomfort when you defecate, if there is blood in your stool, or if you have chronic diarrhea, check with your doctor.

Q. *Since I have become menopausal, I am nearly always constipated unless I use a laxative. Why is this happening and what can I do about it? Is there anything wrong with using laxatives on a regular basis?*

A. Hormonal changes that occur during menopause can cause constipation in some women, similar to the way hormonal changes during pregnancy can cause constipation. The problem with using laxatives on a regular basis is that your body can become dependent on them, and your bowel will literally "forget" how to function without them. In addition, the overuse of laxatives can deplete your body of potassium, an essential mineral that is particularly important for heart function. Long-term use of laxatives can also be irritating to the bowel, and may trigger gastrointestinal problems.

Adding roughage or fiber to your diet, drinking plenty of fluids, and daily exercise are the best ways to treat constipation. Following these simple instructions should eliminate your problem and reduce your need for laxatives.

- Eat at least five fruits or vegetables daily. (Prunes, raspberries, melon, figs, and broccoli are good choices.)
- Eat a high-fiber cereal, such as bran, for breakfast.
- If you cannot get enough fiber through diet alone, use Metamucil, a powdered psyllium supplement daily. (If you become too gassy, cut down on the dose.)
- Drink between six and eight glasses of water daily to soften and bulk stool.
- If necessary, use lactulose syrup. This is an osmotic laxative that is not absorbed into the body and facilitates the entry of water into the colon.
- Exercise every day. At the very minimum, walk between one and two miles daily. Yoga-type exercises that involve squatting are particularly good for stimulating the bowel.

Some cases of constipation are caused by medications. Antidepressants such as Elavil, antihistamines, antihypertensive drugs like calcium channel blockers, and some pain killers are likely culprits. If you are taking any medications on a regular basis that could be causing constipation, talk to your doctor about changing to a different drug.

True constipation is defined as not having a bowel movement for at least three days. If your constipation persists for a week or longer, call your doctor.

Q. Lately, I have been having a problem with passing gas. It is not only uncomfortable, but it is extremely embarrassing. I try to eat enough fiber and avoid spicy foods. What more can I do?

A. Excess gas or flatulence is a common problem among women, especially after menopause. It is caused by the accumulation of gases—including hydrogen, methane, and carbon dioxide in the large intestine—that are produced by so-called good bacteria that help in the digestion of food. In most cases, gas is not a symptom of a medical problem and can be controlled by making changes in your diet. If dietary changes do not solve the problem, however, then you should definitely see your doctor for a thorough examination since chronic gas could also be a sign of gallbladder disease, problems in the digestion of foods such as lactose or fats, or some other gastrointestinal problem. I would try these simple measures first to see if they help.

The right amount of fiber Many of my patients who complain of excess gas are simply too zealous about consuming fiber. Fiber is the cellulose or roughage in food that is indigestible. In the right amounts—about 20 grams daily—fiber can prevent constipation (a condition that can also produce excess gas) and lower cholesterol, and may even prevent cancers of the colon and rectum. In high amounts, fiber can actually irritate the gastrointestinal tract. In particular, I have noticed that many of my patients who complain about gas are using large doses of psyllium powder (Metamucil) to keep their bowels regular. Very often, simply cutting back on the psyllium can relieve the gas problem.

Some forms of fiber are more problematic than others. For example, foods such as broccoli and cauliflower can cause gas in many people and reducing your intake of these foods may help. In addition, legumes (lentils, kidney beans, pinto beans, etc.) contain high quantities of an indigestible carbohydrate that can ferment in the large intestine and cause extreme gassiness. If you eat a lot of legumes, there are products sold over-the-counter (such as Beano) that have been shown to prevent gas when taken with meals. Soaking dried beans for several hours before cooking can also help remove some of the indigestible carbohydrates.

Lactose intolerance In some people, excess gas may be a sign of lactose intolerance: Their bodies do not produce enough of an enzyme called lactase, which is essential for the breakdown of lactose, a sugar found in milk and other dairy products. Many women load up on dairy products because these foods are an excellent source of calcium, a mineral that is needed to prevent osteoporosis. If you are lactose intolerant, you do not have to eliminate dairy products from your diet, but it may be necessary to use special lactose-free products that are now sold in many supermarkets. In addition, you can try a

76

lactase enzyme supplement, which helps to digest the offending sugar. Some supplements come in liquid form that can be mixed into milk; others must be taken during or right after eating a dairy product.

Chew each mouthful Part of the digestion process begins in the mouth when you chew your food, breaking it down into smaller pieces that are more easily assimilated by the body. If you swallow big pieces of food, it will take longer for the food to be digested in the intestine, and the longer it sits in the intestine, the more likely it is to produce gas.

Over-the-counter remedies There are many over-the-counter medications (antacids, antigas) that claim to help keep gas at a minimum. Some contain charcoal, which may absorb gas; others are peppermint-based. (Peppermint is an old-fashioned remedy for gas!) There is no scientific evidence that these medications work, although many people say they help. Some antacids, however, may contain ingredients that are constipating (such as calcium carbonate or aluminum hydroxide), which can create different problems. Another unwanted effect of antacids is that they may impair absorption of medicines: oral estrogen, for example. I would not recommend using these products on a regular basis.

Q. *When I have sex in the missionary position, I find that I pass gas, which is, needless to say, horribly embarrassing. When I told my doctor about this, he joked that I should just "scream to cover the noise." Any better suggestions?*

A. My first suggestion is that you change doctors and hopefully find one who will give you more constructive advice.

As uncomfortable and embarrassing as it may be, it is not unusual for some woman to pass gas during intercourse. If your abdomen is distended with gas, compression during intercourse may well cause it to erupt through the anus, particularly in women with poor muscle tone. Other women may loose air from the vagina during intercourse, which can also be noisy. If you are passing air vaginally, you can try to contract the vaginal muscles more tightly over the penis during sex, which may prevent air from escaping. In addition, I recommend two exercises that can help improve muscle tone in both the anal and vaginal area. You can do these exercises sitting, standing, or lying down as many times a day as you can. You will notice an improvement within a week.

1. Contract the muscles in your anus (as though you were trying not to defecate) and hold for a count of five; then release.
2. Contract the muscles around your vagina and hold for count of five; then slowly relax the muscles.

77

You should also read the answer to the question on constipation in which I discuss methods to reduce excess gas (page 82).

Q. *I was recently diagnosed with a hiatal hernia. How did I get it? What can I do about it?*

A. A hernia is the protrusion of all or part of an organ through a weak spot in the wall of the structure that contains or overlies it. In a hiatal hernia, a portion of the stomach protrudes through the diaphragm, the muscular structure that separates the chest contents from those in the abdomen. Unless the stomach becomes trapped and constricted by the muscle tissue through which it herniates, a hiatal hernia is not life-threatening. Many slip back into position without any treatment.

Many hiatal hernias cause no problems at all. Others coexist with (but do not cause) a defect in the muscular ring at the end of the esophagus that guards the entry into the stomach. When it functions properly, the muscular ring (called the "esophageal sphincter") functions like a one-way valve to prevent partially digested food and stomach acid from regurgitating backward up into the esophagus. The reflux produces burning, belching and chest pain.

We do not know what causes a hiatal hernia. We do know that it is more common in women than in men, and it is most likely to strike during middle age. The discomfort that accompanies a hiatal hernia can be treated in several ways:

Watch your diet. Certain foods are known to aggravate heartburn; they include coffee (even decaffeinated), cola drinks containing caffeine, chocolate, and alcohol. Fatty foods (french fries, fried chicken, etc.) may also trigger symptoms because fat takes longer to be digested in the stomach, thus giving it more time to back up into the esophagus.

Eat frequently and slowly. Eating several small meals throughout the day is better than gorging on two or three big meals. Do not gulp down your food; if you do, it is more likely that you will swallow excess air, which could be irritating.

Sleep with your head raised. The most effective way to do this is to put two telephone books under the top feet of your bed. Simply raising the head and chest with several pillows is insufficient because people change position frequently during normal sleep. Do not lie down within two hours after eating.

Antacids. Over-the-counter antacids or prescription antacids may be helpful in controlling heartburn.

Q. *I have a history of gastrointestinal problems. Although I went from doctor to doctor looking for an answer, enduring some of the most unpleasant tests you can imagine, no one has ever been able to pinpoint my problem. Recently, I was finally diagnosed with irritable bowel syndrome, and instead of offering any medical treatment, my doctor suggested that I see a psychiatrist to help me cope with stress. Huh? I have stomach pain, why should I see a shrink?*

78

A. Irritable bowel syndrome (IBS) is the most common gastrointestinal diagnosis in the United States and is three times more likely to afflict women than men. In reality, IBS is what we call a "wastebasket" diagnosis, meaning it is used only when every other possibility has been ruled out. In fact, there is real confusion in the medical community over what exactly constitutes IBS. Typically, a diagnosis of IBS will be used to cover a wide variety of symptoms ranging from stomach pain of unknown origin to excessive diarrhea and/or constipation to gas, nausea, and painful bowel movements. In women, irritable bowel syndrome is one of the major causes of pelvic pain.

Many GI specialists consider IBS to be more of a disorder of the psyche than of the gut, and refer their patients to psychiatrists. This it's-all-in-the-head attitude may in part stem from the fact that there are no definitive criteria for this problem, and that stress and anxiety may indeed aggravate symptoms. I cannot help but think, however, that, since IBS is a predominantly female problem, many male specialists may be more dismissive of their female patients than of their male patients, and more likely to believe that their problems are psychologically rooted. In fact, I recently saw a disturbing report in which, based on one small study, researchers made the sweeping claim that most women with IBS have a prior history of sexual abuse! Whenever I see a general statement like this one, I am highly skeptical.

Recent studies have shed some light on IBS that may answer some important questions. Based on the latest information, it now appears that IBS is not a psychological problem but a physical one. Researchers believe that people with IBS have a disorder of the nerve supply between the gut and the brain that alters normal pain perception. In other words, they feel pain more intensely. Any physician who has examined a patient with IBS can verify that these patients do appear to experience more pain and discomfort during diagnostic tests of the bowel and rectum than those without this problem. More research needs to be done until we fully unravel the mystery of IBS. For example, we do not fully understand why some people with this problem become constipated and others have diarrhea. Nor do we fully understand what role, if any, stress may play. Until we have all the answers, there are things that patients can do to help themselves feel better.

Medication. Levsin is one of a class of drugs called anticholinergic compounds that lessen the contraction of muscles in the bowel wall. These drugs help to relieve the painful spasms characteristic of IBS.

Control constipation If constipation is a problem, adding fiber and water to the diet can soften stool and promote regular bowel movements.

Control diarrhea Kaopectate or Lomotil are good for this.

Avoid irritating foods Some IBS patients find that certain foods aggravate their symptoms. Keep a food diary for a week to see if you can identify which foods may be causing your problems.

Stress relief I am not saying that IBS patients need psychiatric intervention, but I do believe that learning to control stress may help reduce the severity of symptoms. Biofeedback techniques, meditation, and yoga all help control stress.

Q. For several years I have been plagued with peptic ulcers that seem to get worse when I am under periods of stress. I have taken Zantac periodically, but now it no longer works. My doctor suggested that I go on a course of antibiotics. This does not make any sense to me. Why would antibiotics help me to control stress? Should I do it?

A. Peptic ulcers occur in the lining of the stomach (gastric ulcers) or duodenum (duodenal ulcers) where the usual layer of cells has literally been eaten away and is no longer present. If the erosion continues, it can actually extend into a blood vessel and cause internal bleeding.

One of the symptoms of a peptic ulcer is a burning pain that may radiate upward throughout the entire chest. If the ulcer is in the stomach, the pain appears directly after eating. If it is in the duodenum, the discomfort may take a few hours to appear.

It was once believed that all peptic ulcers were caused by the overproduction of hydrochloric acid (HCl) in the stomach. So the drugs of choice for ulcers were those that blocked the production of hydrochloric acid, such as Zantac and Pepcid. These drugs still help to control the symptoms of the ulcer and, in fact, may be used as short-term therapy, but they do not cure the ulcer.

In the 1980s, two Australian doctors, Barry Marshall and Robin Warren, shook up the medical establishment by reporting that ulcers were actually caused by the H. pylori bacterium and could be cured by a simple course of antibiotics. The medical establishment was initially very skeptical about this claim, but study after study has confirmed that, in most cases, ulcers can indeed by cured by antibiotic therapy. In fact, according to a recent study published in the *Journal of the American Medical Association*, patients taking antibiotics to kill H. pylori are five times less likely to experience a recurrence of their ulcer symptoms than those using acid blockers.

When a patient complains of chronic gastrointestinal pain, most physicians will try a course of medication, usually one that blocks acid production by the parietal cells of the stomach. If the symptoms persist or recur, the patient should have a flexible tube passed through the esophagus into the stomach so that the doctor can see precisely what is the cause of the problem and biopsy the stomach lining for the presence of the H. pylori bacterium. If

H. pylori is found, the treatment consists of a short course of two different antibiotics and bismuth subsalicylate to control the acid output.

If ulcers are caused by a bacterial infection, why do ulcers tend to flare up during stressful periods? There is no question that strong emotion can increase stomach acidity, which would irritate any existing lesions. It is no coincidence that many people find that their ulcers worsen when they are upset. In addition, studies have also shown that extreme stress can dampen the immune system's ability to fight infection. It is possible that the same kind of extreme stress that can increase acid secretions can also hamper the ability of the immune system to stop the overgrowth of H. pylori in the stomach.

Dizziness

Q. *Lately, I have been feeling lightheaded and dizzy, especially when I move my head. It is particularly troublesome in exercise class when I lie down on a mat to do floor exercises. Sometimes, when I stand up, I feel like I'm going to black out. I am quite healthy otherwise, and wonder what could be causing this dizziness?*

A. Dizziness is one of the most common complaints that doctors hear from their patients. In fact, between 5 and 10 percent of all initial visits to general practitioners involve a complaint of dizziness! Dizziness appears to be somewhat more prevalent among women than men, and although it is a common problem among the older population, it can also strike younger women.

Dizziness is a general symptom that could be a sign of numerous problems, only a handful of which would be considered serious. In your case, it sounds to me as if your dizziness is caused by low blood pressure, a condition we call postural or orthostatic hypotension. In this condition, the heart does not pump the blood with enough force to supply the brain adequately, so when you stand up or lie down, you may feel lightheaded for a second or two until the blood reaches the brain. Some people with this problem may find that they feel faint or lightheaded if they jump out of bed too quickly in the morning, or get up too quickly from a chair. Postural hypotension can be easily diagnosed by taking your blood pressure before standing abruptly and then immediately following: The reading should show a sudden drop in pressure. This is not very serious, and can easily be remedied by simply watching your movements. For example, at exercise class, when you are finished with your mat work, do not stand immediately, but rather sit on your mat for a few seconds and then rise to your feet slowly. When you are sitting, contract the muscles in your calves or swing your legs back and forth three or four times before getting up. In the morning, sit on the edge of the bed for thirty seconds before getting up. These simple measures should correct the problem.

There are several other problems that could also cause dizziness. Some of the most well known follow.

Ménière's disease A particularly common form of dizziness is a disturbance of the inner ear called Ménière's disease. The vestibular system of the inner ear and the brain control our sense of balance, but if the inner ear becomes irritated or inflamed, it can throw the sense of balance out of whack. This is what happens in Ménière's disease. The vertigo produced is quite characteristic: In severe cases, even if the patient simply opens her eyes, the room spins and she becomes intensely nauseated. Some patients actually hold on to the bedpost for stability.

We do not know what causes Ménière's disease, although some patients develop the condition after a viral infection or a blow to the head or whiplash injury. In addition to vertigo, many patients with Ménière's disease develop hearing loss and tinnitus, a constant ringing sound in the ear. (In about 10-20 percent of patients, the hearing loss and ringing will also spread to the second ear.) The severity of Ménière's disease varies among patients. Attacks of Ménière's disease can be as infrequent as every few years or as often as several times a month, and can last as long as a few minutes or even a few hours. Treatment includes medication such as meclizine hydrochloride (Antivert), diuretics and antihistamines to dry up any extra fluid in the ear, and even tranquilizers to reduce the feeling of intense motion during attacks. In some cases, ear surgery may be necessary to drain the ear and restore normal pressure. A new treatment called vestibular rehabilitation helps many sufferers. It helps the patient with a defective balancing system learn to rely more on visual clues and input from the nerves in the feet and the legs to overcome vertigo.

Positional vertigo Women with this condition experience dizziness after changing positions or moving their heads. The cause of this problem is unknown: Victims of positional vertigo show no signs of any other physical problem such as an inner ear inflammation or low blood pressure. It is possible, however, that the culprit may be an undetected viral infection. Antivert may help relieve the dizziness. Sometimes patients are instructed to practice the position that causes the dizziness until the balance system can adjust.

Vestibular neuronitis In this disorder, patients suffer from severe vertigo that is often accompanied by nausea and vomiting. The attacks can last for hours or days, and the dizziness and loss of balance can persist for weeks or months. Although the cause of vestibular neuronitis is unknown, it is probably caused by a viral infection of the nerve. Patients who are so impaired that they cannot eat or drink any fluids may need to be hospitalized and put on an IV so they do not dehydrate. Antivert and Valium may help relieve the dizziness.

Stress In some cases, dizziness is a sign of anxiety induced by extreme stress. I recently had a patient who complained that she felt dizzy only when she was away from home in a social situation. A careful physical examination revealed no apparent cause for her dizziness. After talking for a while, she revealed that her husband had leukemia and was not responding to treatment. We agreed that her problem was extreme anxiety; with counseling and anti-depressant medication, her condition improved.

If dizziness is severe or very frequent, you should be examined by your doctor. In rare cases, dizziness could be a sign of a stroke or a slow-growing tumor, two conditions for which prompt treatment is essential. Explain your symptoms as clearly as possible to your doctor: It is important for her to know how long your symptoms last and what seems to trigger them (such as standing up suddenly, a social event, doing knee bends in exercise class, etc.). Your doctor should do a thorough physical examination. Depending on your symptoms, your doctor may want to check your eyes for unusual movements as she changes the position of your head or when warm or cold water is injected into a balloon inserted into your ear. These maneuvers help check on the balance systems in the inner ear and brain stem. She may then refer you to a specialist who may test all the parts of the balance system: eyes, muscles and joints, and inner ear, simultaneously.

Doctors

Q. *The company that I work for has just enrolled its employees in a health maintenance organization and I must now select a primary care physician from a long list of names. How do I pick the doctor who is right for me? What can I expect from my first visit? How can I tell if my new doctor is competent and thorough? (I'm a bit nervous about all of this, although I see a gynecologist every year, the last time I had a complete physical was when I went away to college—ten years ago!)*

A. A primary care physician (or an internist) is a "generalist" who is trained to assess all aspects of your health and function. Unlike your gynecologist, who is a specialist in problems of the female reproductive system, a primary care physician will monitor and evaluate all body systems, from your head to your toes. How do you pick a primary care physician from a "long list of names"? The first step is to narrow clown the list. Here are some things to consider.

Comfort and convenience Before you begin to whittle down the list, you need to ask yourself some important questions: Are you more comfortable with a woman doctor? Do you require a specific location? Do you want a doctor who has office hours during the evening or on weekends? Do you want a doctor who will accommodate you during the lunch hour? These are the types of issues you need to address before making your final selection.

Education and experience Most primary care physicians are board certified in family practice or internal medicine, and you should make sure that your new doctor is board certified in one of these subspecialties. Certification means that your doctor has had extra years of training in an accredited program and has passed a demanding examination to make sure she is ready to deliver competent, state-of-the-art care. Check with your county medical society to see if she is board certified. I also recommend that you ask if the doctor has a faculty appointment at a medical school. In general, a faculty appointment is only made to doctors who have met the strictest educational standards. In addition, these doctors are required to teach at the medical school at least once a year, which helps to keep them current in their field.

To learn even more about your doctor, you can request a physician profile from the American Medical Association in Chicago. The profile will tell you where the physician went to school, where she is licensed to practice medicine, how long she has been in practice, and which, if any, are her specialties. (For the address of the AMA, see Resources, page 223.)

Hospital affiliation A physician may be affiliated with one or more hospitals in which she is allowed to admit patients. Before selecting your primary care physician, you need to know to which hospital your physician can admit patients and if you are satisfied with the resources that are available at that hospital. If it is a hospital that you feel is not up to grade, you may need to find another physician. In addition, if you have a particular problem, such as a heart condition, you may want to select a doctor who is affiliated with a hospital that has a state-of-the-art cardiac care unit.

Emergency procedures How does the physician handle an emergency that may arise after hours? Does she send her patients to the nearest emergency room? Does she provide a twenty-four-hour telephone service? If she is in a group practice, does she refer calls to another physician in her practice? You should ask about office procedures ahead of time so that you do not have any unpleasant surprises.

As conscientious as you may be about making your selection, you never really know how you will feel about a doctor until you meet her face-to-face. You may pick the "perfect" physician in terms of location, credentials, and hospital affiliations only to discover that you do not like her "bedside manner." I do not mean to imply that your doctor has to be your best friend—not at all—but it is critical that you establish some rapport with your physician or

86

you will not be forthcoming with important information. If you should encounter a doctor with whom you feel you cannot talk openly, you should keep looking for another one.

The First Visit

THE FIRST VISIT to a primary care physician or an internist should include a comprehensive examination that will provide your doctor with a baseline of information about all systems of your body. A complete, careful assessment should take at least an hour. Follow-up visits for particular problems will probably not be as thorough or take as long. The comprehensive examination should be repeated at least every two years for a healthy woman under forty and annually after that. Although you may not have any significant disease at the time of your first examination, your relationship with your doctor will last for years; it is important for your doctor to know your general health and function so that she has a reference point for the future.

What should you bring? Patients often ask for their records to be sent to their new doctors, or they bring files filled with information on their first visit. Most of this information might not be necessary, although sometimes an important piece of data is included. Your new doctor will ask for whatever she feels she needs (pieces of essential information, like a previous chest X-ray or mammogram, can always be tracked down), but she will want to gather her own data.

Do bring a list of questions that you may have about your health or other concerns, and make sure these questions are answered before you leave the office. Find out when your doctor takes calls from patients during the day. Most doctors set aside a particular time in which they return calls to patients. (As I noted earlier, more than 10 percent of all women walk out of their doctors' offices without asking important questions that are on their minds. Writing down these questions ahead of time will help you remember what you want to ask.)

Getting to know you When you arrive at your new doctor's office you can expect to be treated in a courteous manner by the office staff. Doctors should be reasonably punctual; you should not have to wait more than fifteen minutes for a physician without a good explanation from the office staff or from the doctor herself. If the waiting room is overflowing with patients, and the common practice of the office is to keep patients waiting for hours on end, it is a sign of either overscheduling or poor organization. Remember that the physician is offering a service for which you are paying, and indifference to patients should not be tolerated.

Be ready to supply the office staff with basic information about yourself at the start of your visit. You may have done this over the telephone, but it is a good idea to bring your insurance information with you. Read over any release forms carefully that make it legal for your doctor to send anything in your chart to insurance companies or other investigative agencies. Ask to see what will be sent. You do not want to give your doctor carte blanche to divulge private information about your life. (For more on the privacy of medical records, see page 97.)

Your first conversation with your new doctor should be in her office while you are still fully clothed—initial interviews that are conducted when the patient is undressed can be awkward for the patient and, I believe, may put her at a decided disadvantage. Many patients in this situation will rush through the interview because they do not feel comfortable enough to ask questions or offer full explanations to their doctor's inquiries. Most primary care doctors today are sensitive enough to conduct the first interview with new patients in their offices. If, however, when you walk into your new doctor's office you are handed a hospital gown and sent to a dressing room, I believe it is your right to ask to talk with the doctor before getting undressed.

During the initial interview, the doctor will take a complete personal and family medical history. The first part of the discussion will usually begin with the reason you are in the physician's office. Doctor's call this part of the interview the "chief complaint." Are you there for a regular checkup, or do you have a specific problem? Depending on your answer, the doctor will then ask for further details of the problem or, if you have no particular concern or symptom, will focus on your overall health.

The next part of the interview is called the "review of symptoms." The doctor will go through all the systems of your body, beginning with your head and neck and proceeding down through your heart to your digestive tract and genitourinary system. She will ask about your allergies, your skin, and your endocrine function, too. This is not only an important part of your first consultation, but it should be repeated once a year during your annual physical. From this discussion, your doctor will often pick up important information about your overall health.

The doctor will then ask questions about your past medical history and will record information about any previous operations, past hospitalizations, accidents, or injuries.

Next, the doctor will ask questions about the health of your immediate family members. She is not prying: It is important to know if there is any history of genetically determined illnesses or early deaths in your family. If your doctor knows that you have a family history of heart disease, cancer, depression, or alcoholism, she can be vigilant about monitoring you for these problems.

Finally, the doctor will take a social history. (I take this part of the patient's story first: I like to know something about my new patient as a person before I begin to talk about her medical problems.) I ask my new patients questions about their education, occupation, personal habits, marriage, schedule, and diet. What a patient is enthusiastic—or discouraged—about often tells me what is important in her life. It forms the basis for a personal relationship between us that is more comprehensive than just knowing about her stomach or gallbladder. It also gives the patient a chance to sit down, relax, and unwind and to answer questions that are not as emotionally charged as those about her health or specific ailments. This part of the interview sets the stage for putting into context the medical details that will he coming next.

If you have any questions for your doctor, now is a good time to ask them. I often advise patients to come prepared with a list of any relevant questions they may have. (By relevant I mean confining the questions to those about your health, not that of your neighbor's, parents', children's, or spouse's health. It is not only a waste of the doctor's time to speculate on the condition of people she has not examined, but by discussing others, you are doing yourself a disservice: This is *your* time; when you should be focusing on *your* health.)

The physical examination After the initial interview comes the physical examination in the examining room. The patient ought to be completely undressed for this, with a gown on and a sheet available on the examining table. Usually, the doctor's assistant will take your "vital signs" (temperature, blood pressure, height, and weight) before the doctor begins her examination.

Many doctors will have a "chaperon" (a nurse or assistant) stay in the examining room throughout the examination, particularly if they are meeting a new patient. Although some patients may find the presence of a second party comforting, others may find it intrusive. Given the intimate nature of these examinations, and the litigious nature of our society, many doctors believe it is important to have a third party present to monitor the proceedings. In my office, my nurse stands behind a screen most of the time so that the patient knows she is there, yet she is not looking in on all the details of the exam.

After your "vital signs" are taken, the doctor will begin the comprehensive examination. She will start by looking at your whole body: She will check your skin for any rashes or moles and examine your bones to make sure they are straight and symmetrical. The doctor will watch you walk to examine your gait and posture and to make an assessment of your general state of development, health, and nutritional status.

She will then focus on particular body parts: assessing your hair, scalp, eyes, ears, nose, mouth, teeth, and tongue. She will look into your eyes with

89

an ophthalmoscope to see the back of your eye; it is a good window to assess the state of your small arteries and it gives a clue to other diseases such as diabetes and high cholesterol. Your vision and hearing will be tested, too.

During the examination of your neck, the doctor will listen to your neck with a stethoscope to pick up any obstructions in your carotid arteries (the arteries feeding blood to the brain). She will feel for any enlarged lymph nodes in your neck and look at your thyroid to make sure it is not enlarged and that there are no lumps in this gland.

A thorough examination of your breasts should follow. The doctor should examine both breasts, your armpits, and the area above your collarbone to make sure there are no suspicious lumps. Some women have asked me why the manual breast examination is needed at all if they get an annual mammogram. A mammogram is not enough to be sure that you do not have a problem. Although it helps to detect early lesions, it may not pick up some of the problems that only a careful examination can reveal. For example, if a woman has heavy breasts, a mammogram may miss a small growth that a careful manual examination would detect.

The doctor proceeds next to your chest, both tapping on your chest (percussion) and listening to it through the stethoscope to see whether your breath is even, or whether there are any unusual sounds that might signify a problem. Your heart examination follows: The doctor places her hand over your heart to feel the quality of the beat and its position, and then listens carefully to all parts of the heart.

The next stop is your abdomen, where the doctor uses her stethoscope to listen to your bowel sounds (they make a characteristic noise) and to listen for narrowing of the large blood vessels that pass through to your legs. Then she will feel for enlarged organs or masses and to see whether you have any points of special tenderness.

Your primary care doctor should be able to do both a pelvic examination and a rectal examination. A Pap smear and if necessary a culture of vaginal secretions are done during this examination. During the rectal examination, your stool is tested for blood, which could be a sign of colon cancer. (In a stool guaiac examination, your doctor puts the stool sample collected from the finger of the examining glove on a specially treated paper and adds a solution to test for blood. If blood is detected, the doctor will refer you for further testing.)

Finally, the doctor will test your neurological status—that is, the function of your nervous system. She will test your mental function by asking such mundane questions as the date and location of her office. She will also test your memory by asking you to remember a list of two or three items that she will later ask you to repeat, and finally, she will have you do some simple calculations. She will test the state of the great nerves of the head that supply the eyes, nose, mouth, face, and neck. Then she will do a general assessment of

90

muscle strength and the reliability of the nerves that help us feel impulses and keep our balance. The function of the cerebellum (the part of the brain that controls balance and small, rapid coordinated movements) is also assessed. Finally, the doctor taps over the major tendons of muscles in your arms and legs with a rubber hammer to test for the state of your reflexes. It is important to document whether or not you have any abnormal movements like a tremor or a problem with balance that could be a sign of a neurological disorder.

At the end of the examination, the doctor or her assistant will draw blood and take a urine sample that will be sent to a laboratory for analysis. The standard tests look at the function of your liver and kidneys, check for diabetes, check your blood for abnormalities in the number of particular types of blood cells, and check the levels of serum fats and thyroid function. The doctor may also recommend tests for special situations (such as estrogen levels for postmenopausal women).

At the end of the examination, the doctor should briefly see you again in her consulting room to explain her findings and to give you her opinion about whether you need treatment or medications. If you are given a prescription for any medication, make sure that you review with your doctor what the medication is and how to take it (at what time, with food or without food, etc.).

A follow-up call is also usual (it might also be a letter, but this is not necessary) to let you know the results of your laboratory data within two or three days following your visit.

If you have any questions about your visit, you should feel free to call your doctor or a member of her staff during the designated telephone hours.

FOLLOW-UP VISITS

FOLLOW-UP VISITS between your annual physicals may be shorter and more to the point, especially if your doctor is "squeezing" you in between other appointments. At these times, it is not unreasonable for your doctor to deal with the particular problem at hand. If, however, there is something you need to discuss with your doctor at greater length, alert the nurse or receptionist when you make the appointment. Be sure to state clearly that you will need extra time with the doctor so that they can schedule the appointment accordingly.

Q. *I met my doctor at a party last week and he asked me out to dinner. I find him very attractive and would like to go out with him, but I feel a bit awkward about seeing him socially. Am I being silly, or should I go?*

A. Under most circumstances, I believe that dating between patients and doctors should be discouraged, particularly if the patient is under the doctor's care for a medical problem. When a woman is ill, she is often in a regressed and vulnerable state; she may see the physician as an omnipotent, powerful, and dominating partner. These relationships can work, but only if, from their inception, the couple recognizes the basic inequality of the relationship, and if the patient does not allow herself to be victimized or manipulated by a person she may consider to be more powerful than herself. In fact, once a social relationship develops between a patient and her doctor, I believe that the patient should get her medical care elsewhere; a romantic partner is no longer objective enough to make the correct decisions in all circumstances.

Q. *Is it true that everything I tell my doctor is strictly confidential?*

A. No, it is not, and this can pose problems for both doctors and their patients. When a doctor takes the Hippocratic oath, she swears to reveal nothing that she learns in the course of her work as a physician. As far as I'm concerned, that means not even revealing the names of your patients to others without a good reason, but this is not always possible or even practical. In reality, state and federal laws may interfere with this confidentiality. For example, in some states, physicians are required to report the names of people with sexually transmitted diseases (such as gonorrhea or syphilis) to the various state boards of health so that those who came into contact with the infected individual can be notified. (In many states, infection with HIV is excluded from this requirement. Because it produces a fatal and contagious disease [AIDS], people infected with HIV may be the object of serious prejudice and discrimination with regard to such things as employment and housing opportunities. Yet even this law can be carried to extremes: Until a recent change in New York State law, doctors were forbidden to disclose whether or not newborns were infected with HIV, and such children had to wait until the ravages of AIDS became apparent to receive treatment.)

There are situations, however, when a patient's right to privacy may be seriously undermined by the indiscriminate disclosure of medical information. A patient's medical records can include some very sensitive material; for example, a patient may tell her doctor about a substance abuse problem (her own or that of a family member), an extramarital affair, an incidence of criminal behavior, or that she is being treated for a psychiatric disorder such as depression. If your doctor is not scrupulous about maintaining confidentiality, such highly personal information can turn up in your insurance file or even in your personnel file at work. For example, some employers closely monitor their employees' medical treatment in an effort to keep insurance costs down. Sometimes, a personnel officer or the company physician may actually ask to see a patient's medical file to verify treatment; if the person photocopying the file is not careful to include only the pertinent medical information, she may send the employer the patient's personal revelations. Under certain circumstances, a physician's records could even be subpoenaed by a court of law and the physician held in contempt of court if she refuses to comply or if she changes anything on the records. Given the relatively easy access to a patient's medical file, patients may hold back important information from their physicians for fear of it becoming public knowledge. Patients have no choice but to protect themselves against unwarranted intrusion: If you are concerned about divulging a confidence to your physician, ask her directly about her feelings on maintaining patient confidentiality and, more important, what concrete steps she has taken to protect patient privacy. A doctor who is conscientious about maintaining her patient's confidences will have instructed her staff on the importance of maintaining patient privacy, particularly when they release information to insurance companies, employers, and other interested parties. If you confide something to your doctor that you do not want broadcast to the rest of the world, I suggest that you give her clear instructions not to write down the sensitive information, particularly if it has no direct bearing on your health. Many doctors these days have two sets of patient files: the written records and the ones they maintain in their heads. Although many groups can lay claim to the written records, the private interaction between a doctor and patient that is not recorded can remain solely between the doctor and the patient.

Douching

Q. *I have always believed that douching was part of good hygiene, but my daughter's doctor told her not to douche. Who's right?*

A. At one time, doctors routinely instructed their female patients to douche; however, that is no longer the case. Studies have shown that there is a higher rate of infection of the reproductive tract among women who douche than among women who do not. At least one study has detected a significant increase in cervical cancer among women who douche more than once a week. There are also a handful of studies that suggest that douching may increase the risk of ectopic or tubal pregnancy.

What remains unanswered by these studies is whether douching itself promotes infection and other problems by altering the normal vaginal environment, or whether women who have problems tend to douche more than those who don't. I personally believe that the latter is true, and that douching per se may not be dangerous, as long as it is not done more than once a week. That is not to say, however, that douching is necessary. Normal hygiene (daily bathing and showering) is all that is required to maintain personal cleanliness. If you do douche, however, I suggest that you avoid using perfumed or prepackaged chemical mixtures, which could not only be irritating but could alter the normal acid concentration of the vagina. Make your own douching solution by mixing two tablespoons of cider vinegar with one quart of warm water. Do not depend on a douche for contraception. It is not effective or dependable. Do not attempt to ward off an infection yourself by douching; in fact, if you do have an infection, douching can spread it. See your doctor for a precise diagnosis before "self-treating."

Exercise

Q. *I am in my mid-fifties and for the first time in my life, I'm seeing signs of "middle-age spread." Although I lead an active life, I have never exercised on a regular basis. Is it too late for exercise to make a difference?*

A. Until recently, conventional wisdom dictated that the human body begins to deteriorate at around age forty-five and there was little to be done about it. It is true that, by about that time, there is a noticeable decline in muscle and an increase in body fat, and with each passing decade the average adult loses up to seven pounds of lean body mass. What was not known, however, is that this decline is not inevitable, and in fact, a rigorous exercise program can prevent and even reverse some of these changes.

We now know that at any age—from nine to ninety—exercise can make a real difference in how you look and feel. And there are solid studies that can prove this, such as the one performed by Dr. Maria Fiatarone at the Hebrew Rehabilitation Center for the Aged, a long-term care facility in Boston. Dr. Fiatarone developed a carefully planned strength training program to counteract muscle weakness for sedentary women and men in their eighties and nineties. Three days a week, for forty-five minutes at a time, the

96

men and women in the study worked out with weights and on exercise training machines under close supervision. At the end of ten weeks, Dr. Fiatarone found an average of 113 percent increase in muscle strength among the study's participants. The exercisers also experienced a 12 percent increase in walking speed and a 28 percent increase in stair climbing power. What I find particularly interesting is the fact that the people who participated in the study also began to take part in more of the recreational and educational activities offered at the home. In sum, the exercise not only improved muscle mass and strength but also had a profound impact on mobility and lifestyle. Think about it: If a ten-week strength training program can have such a dramatic effect on the bodies and minds of women and men in their eighties and nineties, just imagine what it can do for a woman in her fifties or sixties!

There are compelling reasons for women to exercise at any age. First, exercise will certainly help to strengthen and tone your body, and can reduce and even eliminate "middle-age spread." We also know that regular exercise can bolster the immune system, reduce the risk of developing many different forms of cancer, and can even help prevent heart disease and stroke. For women, weight-bearing exercise, such as walking, running, or jogging, can protect against osteoporosis by helping to maintain bone mass and by increasing muscle mass, which can prevent fractures by absorbing the shock of a fall. Whether it is working out at the health club, power walking with a friend, or following an exercise video, regular exercise is essential for good looks and good health.

Eyes

Q. *Recently, I have been waking up in the morning with dry, gritty eyes, which I find to be quite uncomfortable. Why is this happening? Will eyedrops help?*

A. Dry eye is a common condition that is caused when the lacrimal glands (the tear glands) of the eye fail to produce enough moisture for adequate lubrication. Dry eye is not only uncomfortable but can result in injury to the cornea (the transparent covering over the eyeball), which can impair vision, or increase the likelihood of an eye infection. Postmenopausal women have a natural decline in the flow of moisture from the tear ducts, which is a major cause of dry eye. The cause of postmenopausal dry eye is not fully understood. Some researchers believe dry eye is due to the drop in estrogen, while others feel that it is actually caused by a reduction in the production of male hormones. Whatever the cause, many women find that hormone replacement therapy can help relieve their discomfort.

Another issue for postmenopausal women is a change in the geometry of the lower eyelid and the tear duct (the passage that guides tears safely from the eye into the nasopharynx so they don't run down the face). As a result, tears can overflow from the eyes onto the face; I have watched many elderly women rubbing their eyes to wipe away the tears. Sometimes corrective surgery can be quite helpful for this condition.

In younger women, chronic dry eye can be a symptom of an autoimmune disease, which occurs when the body for unknown reasons begins to produce antibodies against its own tissue. Autoimmune diseases are much more likely to strike women than men, which is why some researchers believe that these problems are somehow related to female hormones. Rheumatoid arthritis, lupus, and Sjögren's syndrome are common autoimmune diseases that may cause dry eye. If you have any joint pain, which could be due to arthritis, or suffer from dry mouth (another problem typical of autoimmune diseases), you should consult your doctor. At times, dry eye could be caused by medications such as antihistamines or antidepressants such as Elavil. If you are taking any medication, check with your doctor to see if the drug could be causing your dry eye. Once you discontinue the medication, your eyes should return to normal.

There are several effective treatments for dry eye, some sold over-the-counter, and some available by prescription only. There are many types of artificial tear preparations that are sold without prescription that may offer some relief. If these don't work, your doctor may prescribe stronger preparations, such as steroid eye drops. In some particularly troublesome cases, surgery may be required to close off the tear ducts to preserve whatever moisture your eye produces.

If you live in a very dry house, a humidifier can help retain moisture. Avoid smoky rooms since cigarette smoke will further irritate your eyes. Dry eye can become particularly troublesome in the winter, especially on cold, windy days. If possible, restrict your exposure to cold, and if you must go out, wear sunglasses to protect your eyes. During the summer, be sure to wear goggles when swimming—many people with dry eye find the chlorine in swimming pools irritating.

People with dry eye should avoid contact lenses because there is too great a risk of corneal abrasion (tear) or infection.

Q. *Why do I get dark circles under my eyes when I'm tired? Is it a sign of vitamin deficiency? Is there anything I can do to get rid of them?*

A. Dark circles under the eyes are really an optical illusion created by the way light is reflected off the skin under the eyes; it is not caused by a vitamin deficiency or any other underlying physical condition. Although we associate lack of sleep with dark circles, fatigue is not always the cause. Regardless of how rested they may be, there are people who always have dark circles under their eyes. For some reason, the skin under their eyes is unusually thin and delicate, which means that their blood vessels are closer to the surface. As the blood passes through the vessels, it may give off a darker hue than the rest of the skin on the face, thus producing the dark shadows. For other people, like yourself, the circles only appear when they are fatigued. Why? When you are tired, the skin around the eyes may lose its elasticity and moisture, which can affect the way light is reflected—or rather not reflected—off this area, thus producing the illusion of shadows beneath the eyes. I do not recommend using heavy, deeply colored cover-up creams under the eye, because these attempts to hide the problem may actually call attention to it, or may accentuate under-the-eye wrinkles. The best concealing agent is a sheer, hydrating cream that contains light-reflecting particles. Try a thin film of vaseline for a start: It's a good lubricant and reflects light.

Q. *My mother has glaucoma and my father has cataracts. So far, my eyes are perfect (I'm forty-three) and I want them to stay that way. Are there any vitamins that can save my eyes? What else should I be doing?*

A. Have your eyes checked by a professional annually after age thirty-five. The tension inside your eyeball should be measured carefully to make sure you are not developing increased intraocular pressure (glaucoma), for which you will need special medication. Undetected glaucoma is a cause of blindness and it is something your doctor should be checking, even when you have your annual physical examination, by lightly palpating your closed eye to see if the globe seems to be unusually hard. But this is only an approximation; you need careful measurement with an instrument your ophthalmologist will apply directly to the surface of your anesthetized eye to be sure you don't have early signs of glaucoma.

Cataracts, which are caused by changes in the lens of the eye, result from a number of factors. Among them, some medications (steroids are one), aging, and diabetes can result in damage to the lens of the eye that lead to cataract formation. If the lens becomes so clouded that vision is impaired, surgery with replacement of the lens is the only treatment. Recently, there have been several studies that have shown that antioxidant vitamins (beta-carotene, C, and E) may help to prevent cataracts. Adding foods rich in these vitamins to your diet, or taking vitamin supplements, is a good idea.

Fainting

Q. *Sometimes I faint after eating a very big meal. Why does this happen? Why do some people faint after hearing bad news?*

A. Fainting is the loss of consciousness, or the complete unawareness of the surrounding world and a lack of any response to stimuli. Fainting is caused by an inadequate blood supply to the brain, a condition that can occur for any number of reasons.

Fainting after or even during a big meal is not all that unusual and is caused by the stimulation of the vagus nerve, which is part of the autonomic or automatic nervous system. (This is the system that controls involuntary mechanisms such as blood pressure and the beating of the heart.) When stimulated, the vagus nerve slows the heart rate and causes the blood pressure to fall, both of which impede the flow of blood to the brain. A distended or full stomach can make the vagus nerve fire, which is what results in fainting. There are some people in whom the act of swallowing a large mouthful of food causes a discharge of the vagus nerve, which can cause them to actually pass out at the dinner table. These people may be helped by taking medicine to block the action of the vagus nerve at least a half an hour before they expect to eat.

101

In some cases, it may be necessary to have the vagus nerve cut to relieve symptoms. This is done under general anesthesia in the operating room.

Similarly, a severe emotional shock can also cause the vagus nerve to fire, which is why some people faint upon hearing bad or shocking news. In some women, an orgasm can stimulate the vagus nerve and cause fainting.

If you have to stand still on your feet for a long period of time, you may faint due to poor circulation. When the leg muscles move, they "milk" the blood that collects in the veins back to the heart. When the leg muscles are inactive, the blood begins to pool in the lower part of the body, which reduces the blood flow to the brain. If you have to stand in place without movement for a while (like soldiers on guard at ceremonial posts, for example), remember to flex the muscles of your calves every fifteen minutes or so to help keep blood from pooling in your legs. Failing to do so is one reason soldiers faint at their posts.

Fainting can also be a sign of a disorder of the heart rhythm or an arrhythmia in which the heart beats either too fast or too slow. Some hearts beat so rapidly there is little time for them to relax long enough to fill up with enough blood to supply the body adequately. As a result, the brain is deprived of blood and oxygen, and the individual loses consciousness. On the other hand, some hearts beat so slowly that they do not pump enough blood per unit of time to the brain, and the individual faints. In fact, if the heartbeat is too slow, it may be necessary to install an artificial pacemaker in the chest near the heart. A pacemaker is a small, battery-operated unit that produces electrical impulses that stimulates the heart, causing it to contract, thus ensuring the regular flow of blood throughout the body.

Fainting due to stimulation of the vagus nerve is often preceded by nausea, sweating, anxiety, dizziness, and a sense of fading vision. If you feel faint, do not try to get up immediately—this will only further compromise the flow of blood to the brain. Try to lie flat or put your head between your knees to bring more blood to the brain. One of the commonest mistakes would-be rescuers offer an unconscious patient is to pull them to a sitting or even standing position—the worst idea in the world, because gravity further stresses the brain's blood supply! Loss of feces or urine during fainting, or a bitten tongue, are all signs of a problem more complicated than a simple faint, such as a seizure disorder, and should have the immediate attention of a physician. In fact, any loss of consciousness should be reported to your physician as soon as possible.

Fertility

Q. *I recently heard that women who have taken fertility drugs are at a much higher risk of developing ovarian cancer. With both of my pregnancies, I had difficulty conceiving and needed to take Clomid. When I look at my two wonderful children, I'm happy I did what I did, but given this recent news, I'm also very worried. Is there anything I can do to help protect myself against ovarian cancer? If I get ovarian cancer, can I be cured?*

A. You are referring to a study that was conducted at the University of Washington and the Fred Hutchinson Cancer Center in Seattle in which researchers found that women who took fertility drugs were two and half times more likely to develop ovarian cancer than women in general. Women who took a particular fertility drug known as Clomid (clomiphene) for more than twelve months were at greatest risk. To put this in perspective, this means that instead of a 2 percent lifetime risk of developing ovarian cancer, these women have a 4-5 percent lifetime risk. Although the risk is higher than normal, it is still relatively low. Just compare this to the lifetime risk of developing breast cancer, which is 12 percent. (Other studies, by the way, have found no connection between fertility drugs and an increased incidence of ovarian cancer, so we really need more studies to be sure of the consequences of using drugs to help women conceive.)

Naturally, after this study, many women like yourself who took Clomid were extremely worried, especially since the mortality rate from ovarian cancer is high. Keep in mind, though, that one of the reasons ovarian cancer is often fatal is that it is usually symptomless and, as a result, often diagnosed late, well after the cancer has spread. The earlier the diagnosis, the better the outcome. Since you are at a slightly increased risk of developing ovarian cancer, there are certain precautions you should take to make certain that, if you do develop this disease, it is detected early enough so that it can be treated successfully. As part of your annual physical examination, your doctor should give you a simple blood test called CA 125 assay, which measures a protein in the blood that may be elevated in the event of an ovarian tumor. The test is far from perfect; in fact, it often produces a false positive result, meaning it often is high even when there is no cancer. If, however, the levels of CA 125 are elevated, your physician can follow-up by ordering a transvaginal ultrasound, which can detect any tumors or irregularities in the shape or size of the ovaries. A transvaginal ultrasound (also called a sonogram) is a procedure in which an ultrasound transducer (a small wand) is inserted into the vagina. As sound waves bounce off the tissues and organs, the transducer projects pictures of the inside of the uterus and ovaries onto a monitoring screen. A vaginal ultrasound can reveal any abnormalities including cysts or deposits of fluid that could indicate a problem. I recommend that you have both tests annually to make sure you are cancer-free. Be warned that a transvaginal ultrasound might be a little uncomfortable and discuss this ahead of time with your gynecologist.

In addition to careful medical monitoring, there are other steps that you can take to maintain maximum health. Cutting back on saturated fat—the kind that is found in meat, poultry, and full-fat dairy products—and increasing your intake of green vegetables and carrots may help protect against ovarian cancer. In fact, according to one major study performed at Yale University School of Medicine, the more saturated fat a woman consumes in her lifetime, the greater her risk of developing ovarian cancer. Conversely, the more fruits and vegetables a woman eats, the lower her risk of developing ovarian cancer. Although researchers are not sure why saturated fat would increase the risk of ovarian cancer, some suspect that it may somehow increase the production and circulation of certain potent estrogens that may trigger tumor growth. On the other hand, certain vegetables may have compounds in them that are weak, estrogen-like substances that reduce the body's need to produce more potent forms of estrogen that can promote cancer.

Q. *I'm trying to get pregnant and family members and friends are giving me all kinds of tips. My aunt told me that walking around after intercourse will prevent the sperm from uniting with the egg. Would staying in bed or even doing a headstand after intercourse help move the sperm along?*

A. Lying in bed quietly after intercourse may help the sperm navigate upward and join with the egg. One of the simplest ways to keep the sperm near the cervix after intercourse is to insert a diaphragm after sex and before standing up. This will help keep sperm near the cervix for some hours. A headstand might also push the sperm in the right direction, but using the diaphragm is simpler and the effect is more longer lasting.

I do not want to suggest, however, that pregnancy is not possible unless you resort to these measures. Many women get pregnant whether they stand, sit, walk, or even jog after intercourse. The simple things I recommend may simply help tip the odds in your favor.

Q. *I am unmarried and in my mid-thirties. I'm worried that by the time I meet the right man, I will no longer be able to have children. Is there anything I can do to preserve my fertility?*

A. With more and more women pursuing careers and postponing parenthood, yours is a common concern among women your age and for good reason. There is no question that the ability to conceive and carry a child to term begins to decline once a woman reaches her thirties, and decreases exponentially with each passing year. This is an irrevocable fact of life. Women are born with a finite number of eggs, and as we age, those eggs become fewer and less viable. By the time a woman is forty, it is more difficult to get pregnant, and even if she does, there is a higher chance of miscarriage. There is also a greater risk of having a baby with a genetic problem such as Down syndrome, one of the most common forms of retardation.

Now, for the good news. Despite the odds, the number of women giving birth successfully in their late thirties and even their mid-to late forties is on the rise and many of these women do so with few if any problems. Obstetricians today are more experienced and better skilled in treating older mothers-to-be. Prenatal testing has made it easier to detect problems in utero, and some of these problems can actually be treated before the baby is born. In other cases, the expectant mother is better prepared to deal with the problem after her child is born or she may decide to terminate the pregnancy.

As far as protecting your fertility, there are some simple things you can do to help tip the odds in your favor. I might add that there are also some complicated (and expensive) things that you can do if you are determined to become a mother at any age. Let's begin with the easy things first.

One of the simplest ways to guard against infertility is to protect yourself against infection. Many cases of infertility are a result of residual damage (such as scarred fallopian tubes) and other problems that are caused by "silent" sexually transmitted infections, such as chlamydia, that often go undetected and untreated. In women, these infections are often symptomless and may inflict great harm before they are discovered. Fortunately, sexually transmitted diseases can be prevented. In order to prevent infection, it is essential to have your sexual partner use a latex condom even if you are taking oral contraceptives. It is also a good idea to limit your sexual encounters to people you know are healthy and to practice "safe sex." (For more information on how to prevent sexually transmitted diseases, see the section on AIDS, page 24.) Even if you do not have any noticeable problem, it is a good idea to see your gynecologist once or twice a year so that she can check for any signs of infection. If you detect any change, such as an unusual vaginal discharge, see your doctor immediately. Prompt treatment can wipe out an infection before it can do any irreparable harm. Although preventing infection will not extend your fertile period, it will prevent it from being cut short.

Keep in mind that if you develop any fertility problems when you do try to become pregnant, you have several options to consider. If your eggs are too "old" to be fertilized successfully, motherhood is still a possibility, thanks to in vitro fertilization, a process in which eggs are surgically removed and fertilized outside of the womb. In a variation of this procedure, a donated egg from a younger woman is fertilized and then implanted inside the uterus of the older mother. This procedure has been performed successfully on women of all ages and, in fact, has even made it possible for menopausal women to become mothers with the help of hormone shots throughout their pregnancy.

Women have asked me if it is possible to freeze their eggs when they are young so that they can use them when they are older. Although research is ongoing in this area, this particular procedure is not yet feasible. Recently, researchers have been able to remove an entire ovary from young women undergoing chemotherapy or radiation (which can destroy ovarian function), freeze it, and then reimplant it when the treatment is completed. So far, the only women who have undergone this procedure have been cancer patients of childbearing age. As of this writing, there have been no recorded pregnancies, although doctors are hopeful there will be in the near future. Whether this procedure will be made available to healthy women who are concerned about prolonging their fertile years remains to be seen.

It is possible today to freeze a *fertilized* egg (known as an embryo), which can then be stored indefinitely. The problem with this option is that if you do not have a father in mind, you would have to use donor sperm from a sperm bank, which, for many women, raises some serious practical and ethical questions. What if after storing an embryo, you meet the right man and want to have his children? Do you discard the embryos that you have already fertilized? Do you donate them to someone else? In addition, this procedure can cost thousands of dollars and is not usually covered by insurance.

Q. *My husband and I have been trying to conceive a child for nearly a year, but we have not been successful. To make matters worse, lately I have been under a great deal of stress at work and my periods have not been as regular as they used to be; could stress be making me infertile?*

A. The relationship between stress and infertility is a much misunderstood one and, until recently, has been somewhat of a neglected subject. This was not always the case, and, in fact, at one time stress was considered a major cause of infertility. Years ago, when a couple would have difficulty conceiving, their doctor would typically advise them to relax, take a vacation, and "let nature take its course." Sometimes this advice worked, but if it didn't, medical science had very little else to offer an infertile couple. Today, this approach has fallen out of favor and for good reason. The treatment of infertility is no longer left to chance: Infertility is now regarded as a serious medical problem that can and should be treated aggressively with any number of sophisticated diagnostic techniques and treatment regimes, often with great success.

This is good news for the 15 percent of all couples who will have a problem with infertility—that is, who will be unable to conceive a child after a year of regular sexual intercourse. After a couple has spent a year trying unsuccessfully to get pregnant, a physician will typically advise them to see an infertility specialist for a complete workup to determine what, if anything, is preventing conception. In more than 90 percent of all cases, the inability to conceive will be due to a physical problem in either the man or woman that is often correctable.

Nevertheless, despite the spectacular technological advances that have made it possible to create life in a test tube, many couples will never be able to conceive or carry a pregnancy to term. The inability of technology to "cure" infertility has led some researchers to believe that perhaps there may be other factors involved in infertility that cannot be corrected by fertility drugs or surgery. Maybe, just maybe, those old-fashioned doctors knew something that we did not; perhaps stress does play a role in at least some cases of infertility.

This is not as far-fetched as it sounds, according to Alice Domar, who is a senior scientist at Harvard Medical School's Mind/Body Medical Institute, where she directs a behavioral medicine program for infertile couples at Deaconess Hospital in Boston. Dr. Domar notes that when our bodies are pumping out high levels of stress hormones, it can profoundly affect the levels of other hormones, including those that regulate sexual function. We know, for example, that when some women are under extreme physical or emotional duress, they may stop menstruating. It is as if their bodies are telling them, "Okay, we have to face a tremendous challenge right now, so we don't have the time for luxury functions such as reproduction."

Nevertheless, there are many women who are able to conceive under the most stressful of conditions in the most turbulent of times. Despite near starvation and the constant threat of death, babies were still conceived in concentration camps during World War II and years later in Sarajevo amid continual bombardment by the enemy. Obviously, different people respond to stress in different ways; just as one woman may develop a headache when she is overstressed, and another may be unable to sleep, still another may develop hormonal problems that interfere with reproduction.

Dr. Domar also notes that even when infertility is purely physical in origin, the process of being diagnosed with infertility and undergoing what can often be arduous treatments can also be very stressful. It can be difficult to distinguish between people who are suffering fertility problems because of stress and those who are continuing to experience infertility because they are stressed out by their inability to conceive. "It's a chicken or the egg kind of question. Medical tests and high-tech in vitro treatments can be very stressful and that might very well somehow affect a woman's body."

This is not to suggest that we should turn back the clock and treat infertility as purely an emotional issue. But given the close relationship between stress and infertility, I would advise anyone who is undergoing treatment for infertility to ask her doctor to refer her to a stress management program. I am not suggesting that learning stress management techniques will guarantee a pregnancy, but at the very least it could help you better cope with a particularly difficult time of life.

Fibroid Tumors

Q. *Five years ago, I had several fibroid tumors removed from my uterus. I was fine for a while, but the fibroids have grown back and I am miserable. I have very heavy periods and am quite uncomfortable. My doctor told me that there is no guarantee that if I have the fibroids removed again, that they will not grow back. He also said that the fibroids may shrink when I become menopausal, and maybe I should consider waiting a bit before doing anything. (I'm forty-eight years old, and will probably be menopausal within a few years.) He also said that he could put me on a drug that may shrink the fibroids, but it would trigger an early menopause and there were some side effects that did not sound too appealing. Frankly, I'm not sure what to do. Should I take the drugs, or have more surgery to remove the fibroids? Should I consider a hysterectomy? Since I do not want any more children, is there any reason not to consider a hysterectomy? Do I have any other options?*

A. Until recently, it was very common for women with fibroids to be told that they had no option other than a hysterectomy in which the entire uterus is removed. In fact, there were so many hysterectomies being performed for fibroid tumors—a condition that is nearly always benign—that women's groups as well as many physicians began to question whether much of this surgery was necessary. Although this controversy led to a revolution in the way fibroids are treated, it also gave women what may appear to be a bewildering array of choices, with no perfect solution. It sounds to me as if your doctor is proceeding with caution; however, I can understand your confusion and frustration at having to make such a difficult decision. Here are the facts you need to know in order to make the best choice for you.

Fibroids are benign growths or tumors that grow in the walls of the uterus. Some are completely within the wall, but others involve the uterine lining ("submucous" fibroids) and cause excessive uterine bleeding. In 3 out of 1,000 cases, fibroids degenerate into malignant tumors. The cause of the disorder is unknown, but it does have a genetic component in that it tends to run in families. Fibroids are one of the most common gynecological problems, and occur in about 1 out of 4 women between the ages of thirty and fifty. These tumors can be very tiny, or they can grow to the size of a grapefruit, stretching the uterus as much as it would during the last stages of pregnancy. A woman can have dozens of small fibroids, or merely one or two large ones. If fibroids are small and produce no symptoms, you may not even know that you have them. If, however, the fibroids grow, they can cause unpleasant symptoms such as extra heavy and frequent menstrual periods, which can cause severe anemia, abdominal pain, and pain during intercourse. If the fibroids grow in the wrong place, they can actually interfere with other organ systems. For example, as the uterus stretches, it can push the intestines upwards, changing the shape of the abdomen. If the tumor pushes on the pelvic nerves, it can cause hip or back pain. If the tumor presses down on the bladder, it can cause a constant desire to urinate. During pregnancy, fibroids may compete with the embryo for space and blood supply in the uterus, and can cause a miscarriage or premature delivery.

Fibroids may be detected during a routine pelvic exam; the diagnosis can be confirmed with a ultrasound scan that can usually distinguish a malignant tumor from a benign one.

If fibroids are slow-growing and are not causing any discomfort, there is no reason to do anything about them other than to check them during your annual physical for signs of rapid or abnormal growth. The one exception to this rule would be if the fibroids are growing in such a way that they are blocking the doctor's ability to feel the ovaries during a pelvic examination, or to get a good view of the ovaries during an ultrasound. The risk of ovarian cancer increases in women over forty, and it is imperative that your doctor be able to at least palpate the ovaries during your annual examination.

In about 25 percent of all cases of fibroid tumors, women will not experience any discomfort. If a woman is having excessive bleeding, is in pain, develops severe anemia from bleeding, or is very uncomfortable in other ways (for example, the tumor is pushing on the bladder so hard that she is having trouble urinating), her physician will recommend more aggressive treatment. Depending on any number of factors, the following treatment options will be considered.

Drug therapy Estrogen can stimulate the growth of fibroid tumors. Therefore, it is possible to shrink tumors by using a class of drugs that block the body's production of estrogen. These drugs are called GnRH antagonists (Lupron is the one most commonly used) and can be given by monthly injection or twice daily via a nasal spray. Although GnRH antagonists do reduce the size of tumors within two or three months, they have some significant shortcomings. First, they induce an artificial menopause, and as a result, women on these drugs may experience hot flashes, night sweats, depression, and other menopausal symptoms. Second, the effect is not permanent. Women are usually not advised to stay on this drug for more than six months, and when it is discontinued, the tumors will eventually grow back to their full size. Two types of patients can benefit from this treatment: If you are close to menopause, it may be possible to stave off surgery by shrinking the tumors until you are actually in true menopause, when fibroids shrink on their own due to failing estrogen levels. If you have very large tumors, it may be advisable to take Lupron prior to surgery to shrink the tumors so they are easier to remove.

Myomectomy A myomectomy is a limited surgical procedure in which only the fibroid tumors are removed and the rest of the uterus remains intact. Depending on the location and the size of the tumors, it is not always possible to perform the myomectomy vaginally, and an abdominal incision may be necessary. Recovery then takes longer. In some cases, the surgeon could minimize the size of the abdominal incision by using a laparoscope, a tiny instrument with a light and a camera on the end that is inserted through the belly button and transmits an enlarged image of the internal organs on a TV monitor. Guided by the video image, the surgeon can then make another small insertion near the belly button and remove the fibroids using long-handled surgical instruments.

If a fibroid is outside of the uterus near the cervix, the surgeon may be able to use a hysteroscope, a small telescopic instrument that can be inserted through the vagina and the cervix so that she can examine the uterus without making a major incision. In a very new procedure, the surgeon may be able to burn off or cauterize the tumor using a laser device that can be attached to the hysteroscope. In some cases, the surgeon may use a resectoscope, an instrument that sends electric current through the tumors and destroys them. Although there is risk that the surgery could injure or scar the uterus, which

111

is a concern if you are contemplating a future pregnancy, or that there could be excessive bleeding, in the hands of a skilled surgeon, myomectomy is usually safe and effective. Myomectomy is typically performed on an outpatient basis, which means the patient can go home the same day as the procedure.

The problem with myomectomy is that it is often temporary: As long as there is a uterus, fibroid tumors can grow back. In fact, they will return in about 25 percent of all cases within five years. When the tumors return, your surgeon may repeat a myomectomy. However, multiple myomectomies can lead to complications such as excessive scar tissue, which can actually block the passage of food and waste material through the intestine. If a woman is close to menopause as you are, it may make sense to have a second or even third myomectomy because in all likelihood, it will be your last. Myomectomy is also the treatment of choice for women who want to retain their uterus to have children.

Hysterectomy Hysterectomy is the second most commonly performed surgery in the United States (only cesarean sections are performed more often). About one third of all hysterectomies, some 200,000 annually, are performed for fibroid tumors. A hysterectomy may be required for women who have had multiple myomectomies or for whom there is no other way to remove the fibroids, and there is a compelling reason to do so. For example, if the fibroid tumors are extremely large or so rich in blood supply that hemorrhage during a myomectomy is a real risk, a hysterectomy may be the only option. If hysterectomy is a medical necessity, the physician should try to save the ovaries. *You should know, however, that the ovaries fail to function in a significant percentage of women* immediately after hysterectomy. Almost 50 percent of women who have had a simple hysterectomy (which left her ovaries in) will reach menopause within three years of the surgery. We do not know all the functions of the uterus, and it may well have some supportive role for ovarian function that prevents premature ovarian failure. Most physicians believe that ovarian failure after a hysterectomy is due to a compromised blood supply to those organs as a result of the surgery. I think it may be more complicated than that, and there may be a real need for an intact uterus to preserve good ovarian function for a normal period of a woman's life span.

For these reasons, when a surgeon recommends a hysterectomy, it is important to get a second opinion to see if more conservative treatment is viable. Many women mistakenly believe that after the childbearing years, the uterus is a "useless" organ. This simply is not true. Even when the ovaries are spared, women face a significant risk of premature menopause after a hysterectomy.

Premature menopause is a serious risk factor for coronary artery disease (CAD), and any woman who experiences this should discuss estrogen replacement with her physician, taking estrogen after a premature menopause (before the age of forty) eliminates the increased risk for CAD. In fact, according to one recent study, women who undergo premenopausal hysterectomies have a threefold incidence of CAD for their entire lives.

Hysterectomy can have other unpleasant side effects, including vaginal shortening due to scarring, which can cause pain during intercourse and even urinary tract problems. Loss of the uterus also eliminates both cervical movement during penile thrusting and uterine contractions during orgasm—important components of sexual pleasure for some women. On the other hand, others report that not having a uterus eliminates the need to use contraception so that sexual activity is much more pleasurable.

Hysterectomy for fibroid tumors should only be done as a last resort, and only after every other option has been seriously considered.

Hair

Q. *I'm a young woman (twenty-nine), and I've recently noticed that I'm losing my hair. It is coming out in clumps on my hairbrush, and although I am still far from bald, my hair is a lot thinner than it used to be. Can anything help?*

A. There are different times in a woman's life when she may be troubled by hair loss. The period immediately following childbirth is one of them. During the postpartum period, it is common for hair to begin to thin out and even to lose some of its curl and body. Once hormone levels stabilize, normal hair growth usually resumes within a few months. After menopause, many women may notice that their hair is thinner and finer than it used to be. In your case, however, I suspect that there is an underlying physical problem that may be causing your hair to fall out.

The most common cause of hair loss in women is called androgenetic alopecia, which is due to the effect of male hormones or androgens on the hair follicles, which are located at the root of the hair. Why androgens cause hair to fall out is still a mystery, although some experts believe that male hormones thwart hair growth by shrinking the hair follicle. As its name implies, androgenetic alopecia is believed to be in part hereditary. In some but not all cases, women with this problem have higher than normal levels of circulating andro-gens. Once normal hormone levels are restored, further hair loss can usually be averted. Some women with androgenetic alopecia have normal levels of male hormones, but researchers suspect that for some reason, their hair follicles are very susceptible to even low levels of androgens, thus causing the hair loss.

There is only one FDA-approved treatment to combat hair loss: minoxi-dil, a drug that was originally developed as a medication to lower high blood pressure. Applied directly to the scalp, minoxidil—marketed under the name Rogaine—has been shown to slow down hair loss and stimulate the growth of new hair in some patients. It is also possible that a completely different type of hormonal imbalance could be causing your hair to fall out. For example, an underactive thyroid, a condition shared by more than 10 million American women, can cause hair loss. The thyroid gland sits at the base of the neck and secretes hormones that control metabolism. If you feel depressed, are unusu-ally tired, or are having particularly heavy and frequent menstrual periods; it could be a sign of a sluggish thyroid. Fortunately, this condition is easy to treat with a synthetic thyroid hormone. Once the hormone kicks in, your hair will begin to grow back.

Patchy bald spots on the scalp could be due to a condition called alopecia areata, the exact cause of which is not known, although researchers suspect that it may be due to a virus, an autoimmune disease, or both. There are many treatments for this problem including steroid injections and antiviral drugs. Minoxidil is also effective for some people with this type of baldness.

In some cases, hair loss may be a result of a scalp infection, which can be caused by bacteria or fungi. If your physician suspects an infection may be the culprit, she may biopsy a tiny piece of scalp tissue to determine the cause of the infection. Antibiotics or antifungal medication may be prescribed to clear up the infection.

It is well known that the strong chemotherapy treatments used to fight cancer can cause hair loss, but what is a lesser known fact is that many other commonly used medications can cause hair to fall out, including birth control pills, antidepressants, blood thinners, and medicines used to treat gout. If you are taking any medicine, check with your physician to see if it could be caus-ing your problem. Other factors that could also contribute to hair loss include poor diet, excessive stress, or an iron deficiency. Hair loss is not just a cos-metic concern, it could be a sign of a physical problem, which more often than not can be successfully treated. In extremely rare cases, it could even be a sign of a tumor of the adrenal glands or ovaries. This is why I urge you to bring this matter up with your doctor.

A simple and often overlooked cause of patchy or localized baldness is too much traction on the hair on that part of the scalp. A patient of mine secured her heavy hair in a barrette on top of her head, always placing it in the same spot. She even ignored the pain that sometimes occurred because the barrette pulled on the anchoring hair. Finally she noticed she was losing hair in that area of her scalp and changed the location of her barrette.

Some patients who are severely emotionally disturbed pull out their own hair. Others "twirl" or twist the same strand of hair in a ticlike habit that eventually causes damage to the hair follicles. Some of these people also pick at their own skin so severely that they develop bleeding, scabbed lesions to which they return as soon as a new scab has formed. These habits often improve or disappear with psychotropic medication, particularly the serotonin reuptake inhibitors like fluoxetine (Prozac).

There are, of course, processes for hair transplantation, when small segments of the patient's own scalp (with hair intact) are relocated to the balding area of her head. This process often produces a "spotty" or patchy appearance to the newly festooned area, and may require creative hairstyling to cover gaps, Another technique is hair weaving, which attaches strands of hair to existing hairs already rooted in the patient's head. This is another way to "thicken" hair in an area where growth is sparse.

Q. *Can using a hair dryer every day damage my hair?*

A. If properly used, a hair dryer should not damage hair. Be sure to hold the hair dryer several inches away from the scalp and never use the dryer on its highest temperature. A very hot dryer held too close to the scalp can actually damage the hair follicle and cause permanent baldness. I wince when I watch hair being "blow-dried" in a salon, when the operator combines very hot dryers held close to the scalp with such vigorous pulling of the hair with the brush that the client's head is pulled back by the force of the traction! Personally, I have my own hair shampooed and cut when necessary, and pass on the "blow-dry" component of the operation unless I know the operator will be gentle and not try to use an acetylene torch to hurry the process along!

Q. *Are hair dyes safe? Can they cause cancer?*

A. About one third of all American women use permanent hair dyes, and through the years, there has been debate over whether the chemicals used in hair dye are carcinogenic. In particular, two compounds formerly used in dark hair dyes—4 MMPD or 4 MMPD sulfate—were shown to cause tumors in laboratory animals. Although manufacturers are no longer using these chemicals, there is concern that the new ones being used may pose potential problems because they have not undergone FDA testing. In fact, some consumer groups have been lobbying to have these chemicals banned until they have been thoroughly tested. Before you panic, however, I want to reassure you that two recent, large-scale studies have generally confirmed the safety of hair dyes. The first study, published in the *Journal of the National Cancer Institute* (May 1995), involved half a million women who used permanent hair dyes. Researchers found that even women who had used hair dyes for more than two decades did not have an increased risk of breast, stomach, lung, or other cancers. The only exception was that women who had used black hair dyes for more than twenty years had a slightly increased risk of non-Hodgkin's lymphoma and multiple myeloma, two rare forms of cancer. Another study, which was published several months later (October 1995) in the *Journal of the National Cancer Institute*, involved an investigation of about 100,000 registered nurses by researchers at the Harvard School of Public Health. Unlike the first study, the Nurses' Study did not find any link between the use of hair dyes of any type and an increased risk of any forms of cancer.

Based on these studies, I think it is safe to assume that any hair dye on the market is safe to use. If you are still concerned about using any chemicals on your hair, I recommend that you ask your hairdresser about a natural product called henna, which is basically a vegetable dye. Henna can highlight hair and cover gray, but it is not permanent and needs to be reapplied every six to eight weeks.

Q. *Can an emotional shock cause hair to turn gray overnight?*

A. Not exactly. Severe stress can wreak havoc on a woman's body; it can stop ovulatory function, diminish appetite, depress immune function, and accelerate aging. Although it is not possible for hair to literally turn gray overnight, stress can accelerate both hair loss and loss of color.

Malnutrition can cause hair to fall out and to lose its natural color. After a long period of illness and/or depression, when patients have not had adequate food intake, this is not uncommon. The hair regrows and even regains its normal color in many cases when vitamin supplements and proper feeding are introduced.

Q. *What can I do about severe dandruff?. Over-the-counter shampoos do nothing. Should I stop using my hair dryer?*

A. Dandruff (also called seborrheic dermatitis) is the result of an extremely dry and often inflamed scalp, and is very often a hereditary condition. It is not caused by using a hair dryer, although excessive use of a very hot dryer may exacerbate the condition.

117

Most dandruff shampoos contain the same active ingredients (tar, selenium sulfide, zinc, or a combination thereof) but in varying strengths. The products that are sold over-the-counter are the weakest, and if they do not work for you, your doctor can prescribe a stronger solution. Usually, within a few weeks, a prescription product will show dramatic results if it is used on a regular basis. If, however, a prescription shampoo does not work, your doctor will either increase the strength of the prescription, or increase the duration of the amount of time that you use the product. For example, there are several highly effective treatments for dandruff that require that you leave the solution on overnight. If you are plagued with bad dandruff, talk to your doctor about your treatment options.

Q. *My hair is full of split ends. Are there any shampoos that can help damaged hair? What about vitamin treatments? Can anything help my hair grow faster?*

A. A split end is a sign that the hair cuticle—the outer layer of the hair shaft—is damaged and it is one of the most common hair problems. There is no evidence that vitamins either applied to hair or taken internally can affect hair unless you are suffering from a severe malnutrition, which is not common in the developed world. Protein, however, is one supplement that may help when applied to hair because the hair shaft itself is made primarily of protein. According to dermatologist Mary Gail Mercurio, a hair specialist at Columbia Center for Women's Health, protein-containing shampoos and conditioners can penetrate through the cuticle and may help to smooth out the split end, giving hair a shinier, more even appearance. One of the most common proteins used is keratin, but according to Dr. Mercurio, most any protein will do.

A protein treatment, however, may not be good for very fine hair because it may weigh it down and make it look limp and less fluffy. Protein does work well as a conditioner for thicker, coarser hair.

Finally, hair grows on average one-half inch a month or six inches a year, and there is nothing that can speed it up.

Q. *Since I have become menopausal, I have begun growing hair in places where have I don't want it (under my chin and my nostrils) and losing it in places where I do want it (my head and pubic area). What's going on?*

A. Nothing abnormal, I assure you. The loss of body hair after menopause is a normal and, in fact, welcome event by many women who are delighted by the fact that they no longer have to shave their legs. It is also common for the pubic hair to thin out and to lose its curl. Interestingly, this is not affected by estrogen replacement: Pubic hair remains thinned and straight. Very often,

118

the hair on the head will also thin out after menopause. However, since the hair loss is usually evenly distributed throughout the scalp, it is usually not very noticeable.

What is troublesome to many women is the fact that, after menopause, there can be a spurt in hair growth on the chin and nose. This occurs because as estrogen production by the ovaries falls off, the male hormones women normally produce are unopposed by an adequate amount of "female" hormones and hair growth begins on androgen (testosterone) sensitive sites of the body. Hormone replacement therapy may help prevent some of this unwanted hair growth. If you are not taking replacement estrogen, however, you can have the hair removed. I recommend that you have this done by a qualified electrologist. (Ask your dermatologist to recommend one.) Do not wax unwanted hair; it can produce unsightly infection of the hair follicles and even cause new hair to be trapped within the epidermis.

Headaches

Q. *I suffer from severe headaches before my menstrual period. What is causing these headaches and what can I do about them?*

A. What you are describing is a classic premenstrual headache, which is caused by hormonal shifts. Prior to menstruation, levels of estrogen drop and women often suffer from what doctors call vasomotor instability: vessels constrict more easily than usual, including the vessels in the brain and the coronary arteries.

When estrogen levels are low, so are levels of a hormone called serotonin, which is produced by the brain. Although we don't know precisely how or why, low levels of serotonin are believed to promote headache pain, perhaps by somehow reducing the level of effectiveness of endorphins, the natural painkillers that are produced by the brain. In fact, we know that serotonin levels are consistently lower in patients having tension or migraine headaches, a particular type of throbbing, painful headache that occurs on one side of the head (see the next answer). Women in particular are prone to migraine headaches, especially around the time of their periods. In addition, women who are taking birth control pills or who are on hormone replacement therapy (HRT) are also more likely to develop headaches during the time of the month when they are taken off estrogen. (This is why some physician-experts in HRT recommend that estrogen *never* be interrupted, and that the patient take it 365 days a year.)

When you feel a headache coming on, the best thing to do is to try to sleep; sleeping slows down the metabolism of serotonin, thus relieving the headache. Over-the-counter nonsteroidal anti-inflammatory medications such as aspirin, naproxen sodium, and ibuprofen may also help. These drugs block the production or action of hormones called prostaglandins, which promote muscle contraction and during menstruation can aggravate menstrual cramps. If your headaches are very painful, your doctor can prescribe any number of medications that can prevent or lessen the severity of the headaches including sumatriptan, which enhances the action of serotonin, and ergotamine and beta-blockers, both of which dilate blood vessels.

Q. *I don't get headaches often, but when I do, they are very painful. I get very sick from them and often throw up. My mother thinks I have migraine headaches and that I should see a doctor. Could she be right? Are migraine headaches serious?*

A. Your mother may be right. Migraine headaches are very common among women (women are three times more likely to get migraines than men) and are often accompanied by nausea and vomiting. The typical migraine is often described by patients as a "throbbing" headache, usually causing pain on one side of the head. There are two types of migraines: classic and common. The main difference between a classic and a common migraine is that classic migraine sufferers experience what is known as an aura, which is a characteristic and consistent phenomenon that warns a headache is on the way. Most aura are visual—that is, the sufferer sees flashes of bright light (called scotomata), often in a geometric pattern. The aura is usually but not always followed by a headache. In most cases, the aura disappears within an hour or two; however, for some people, the aura may last for days or even weeks. Classic migraine symptoms can also mimic the symptoms of a stroke, including speech loss, weakness on one side of the body, or tingling or numbness in the face, arms, or hands. (If you experience any of the above symptoms, you should see a doctor to decide whether you are having a migraine or a more serious problem like a stroke.)

A common migraine, which, as its name implies, is the most typical kind, is characterized by a painful headache that is more severe and longer in duration than the average headache. In fact, it is not unusual for a migraine to last up to three days. People who get common migraines do not experience the pre-headache aura, but many do complain of feeling unusually tired, unable to concentrate, and may even experience mood changes. In order to be classified as a common migraine, the headache must also be accompanied by two of the following symptoms: nausea, pain on only one side of the head, pain that is so severe that it prevents normal activity, or pain that is brought about or worsened by normal physical activity. Once a migraine is over, the pain disappears, but many patients complain of feeling exhausted and completely drained.

As many as 15 percent of all women may experience migraine-type headaches. Migraines are not considered serious medical problems unless they are so debilitating that the headaches are preventing you from leading a normal life. If your headaches are infrequent, and you can manage them on your own with over-the-counter painkillers, there is no reason to see a doctor *unless they are of recent onset.* Any new, persistent headache deserves evaluation, and your doctor should do a complete physical examination and take a careful history to be sure the headache is not due to a more serious problem. Another reason to get your doctor's help is for severe pain, particularly if you are experiencing it for the first time. Migraines are so common these days that most doctors have had some experience in treating them. If, however, your problem is particularly complicated, your doctor may refer you to a neurologist or to a special headache clinic staffed by physicians trained in state-of-the-art treatments. If your doctor tells you that there is little to be done for your headaches, it is a sign that she is not up on the latest treatments, and it is then advisable to consult with a specialist.

There are several prescription medications that have been shown to be effective against migraines. They include:

- NSAIDs: Start with simpler, over-the-counter medications like Advil or Aleve; your doctor can write a prescription for other types of nonsteroidal medications if these don't work.
- Sumatriptan: This drug enhances the action of serotonin, a compound produced by the brain, which is believed to be involved in pain control. Patients had to take it by a self-administered injection; now an oral form of the drug is available.
- Vasoconstrictors: Both ergotamine and beta-blockers (which are normally used to control high blood pressure) relieve headache pain. These are taken orally. Ergotamine is used only to abort an attack, while beta-blockading medications are needed on a chronic, everyday basis.
- Butorphanol: A potent pain killer, this drug is available in a nasal spray, which is faster acting than drugs consumed orally.

Very often, if patients use these medications at the onset of the headache, or when they feel a headache is imminent, they may be able to ward it off entirely. In other cases, these drugs may only lessen the severity and reduce the duration of the headache.

When you feel a migraine headache coming on, try lying down in a dark, quiet room. Avoid bright lights, television screens, or computer screens, which could irritate your condition. Some migraine sufferers find that a cup of peppermint tea or a glass of ginger ale can relieve the nausea and sick feeling.

Q. *I wake up with a headache every morning and need to take some kind of painkiller like aspirin or acetaminophen. If I try to skip a day, the headache comes back. Have I become addicted to painkillers?*

A. It sounds to me as if you are experiencing what are known as "rebound headaches," which occur in people who, like yourself, overuse analgesic medication. Some experts believe that rebound headaches occur because the body builds up a tolerance to the medication, thus requiring more and more medicine to achieve the same effect. Others believe that the continual use of artificial painkillers actually dampens the brain's ability to produce its own natural painkillers, thus triggering headaches. One way to cure your problem is to discontinue the use of all analgesics until your body straightens itself out, in other words, going cold turkey. During your recovery time, you may experience more headaches, nausea, and even stomach upset, which can be quite uncomfortable. If going cold turkey doesn't sound appealing, you can also gradually cut down on the use of medication, which may minimize some of the unpleasant side effects. Whatever you decide to do, I recommend that you talk to your doctor first to determine which approach is best for you.

Although it is rare, morning headaches that clear up later in the day can be a sign of high blood pressure. If you have not had your blood pressure checked recently by your physician, you should do so.

Q. *My problem is a variation of the old joke "Not tonight, I have a headache." I get a headache after having sex. What can I do about this?*

A. Some women and men get terrible headaches after having an orgasm. Whatever the cause, the anticipation of a miserable headache after sex can make the experience more of an ordeal than a pleasure. Fortunately, two different types of medication beta-blockers and calcium channel blockers—can help to prevent after-sex headaches. Since you will need a prescription for either one of these drugs, you should talk to your doctor about your problem.

Q. *Help during the workweek I am fine, but nearly every weekend I am plagued by dreadful headaches. Why would this be happening? What can I do to stop it?*

A. Yours is a very common complaint—so common, in fact, that there is even a name for this particular type of headache. It is called a letdown or relaxation headache because, as its name implies, it typically occurs after a particularly stressful event. In your case, you are probably under a great deal of pressure during the week and once you begin to unwind for the weekend, your reward for a hard week's work is a pounding headache. No one knows precisely why this happens, although there are some reasonable theories. When you are under stress, your body is pumping out high levels of certain types of hormones. Your muscles are tense, your blood vessels narrow. Once the stress has passed, the level of stress hormones drops, thus relaxing the muscles, which in turn causes the blood vessels in the head to dilate. This in turn may cause swelling of the blood vessel wall, which irritates the nerves in and around the vessels, which produce the pain that we experience as a headache. Your best defense against the weekend headache is to learn how to control stress during the week.

There are other factors, however, that could also be causing your weekend misery. For example, when one of my patients complained of weekend headaches, I urged her to keep a diary tracking her activities from Friday night through Sunday to see what, if anything, she was doing differently on the weekends than during the week. From her diary, t learned that on Friday nights she always visited her mother-in-law, with whom she had a strained relationship. To make the visit more bearable, my patient—who was normally a teetotaler—would down two glasses of Scotch and soda during the course of the evening. The headache that she was experiencing the next day was actually a hangover. Once she stopped her Friday night drinking, the headaches disappeared.

Anyone who has weekend headaches should examine whether some change in activity could be triggering the headaches. Things to consider include:

Sleep patterns If you sleep later on weekend mornings than during the week, and therefore are eating breakfast later, your headaches could be from low blood sugar. Try waking up earlier and having something to eat, and then going back to sleep. If you typically need several cups of coffee on a weekday morning to get going, and you are sleeping later than usual, your headaches may be due to caffeine withdrawal. Studies have shown that when denied caffeine, caffeine users can develop symptoms of withdrawal, including headache, nausea, cramps, and the inability to concentrate.

Medication Do you smoke marijuana or take Valium or other sedatives to ease into the weekend? If you do, these drugs could produce a "hangover" headache.

Food and drink Do you eat different foods on the weekend than during the week? Some preservatives and flavorings in foods can cause headaches in susceptible people, including monosodium glutamate, which is often used in Asian cuisine, and sulfates, which may be sprayed on produce in salad bars and are also an ingredient in wine. Chemicals found in chicken livers, chocolate, herring, and aged cheese as well as too much caffeine can also cause headaches in susceptible people. Ice cream or cold drinks can also trigger headaches. Obviously, if you are imbibing more on the weekends than during the week, your headaches are probably old-fashioned hangovers.

Stress Some people find the office a stressful place, but others may find it more stressful to be at home, particularly if there is tension between you and other family members. Dealing with the stressful situation is the best way to eliminate the headaches.

Chemicals If you tend your garden on the weekends, you may be using fertilizer or some other chemicals that could be causing your headaches. If you paint on the weekends or putter around the house, you may be exposing yourself to solvents like benzine or turpentine, spray adhesives, rubber cement, and other chemicals that give off fumes that could be triggering your headaches.

Other factors If you have a country house, you may be using a space heater on the weekends that is contaminating the air with carbon monoxide, which can trigger a headache.

It may require some thought and investigation on your part, but once you identify the cause of your headaches, you can take positive steps to control them.

Q. *Every few weeks I get a really terrible headache for no apparent reason. I'm worried that I have a brain tumor. Am I being ridiculous or could I really have a tumor?*

A. I cannot tell you how many of my patients who suffer from headaches have asked the same question. In reality, a headache is rarely the first sign of a brain tumor (less than .05 percent of all brain tumors present as severe headaches). Think about it: Forty-two million Americans seek medical help for headaches each year; yet only 11,000 cases of brain tumors are diagnosed annually. You don't need a Ph.D. in mathematics to figure out that the vast majority of headaches are caused by things other than tumors.

Other symptoms, along with a headache, could be signs of a tumor—or any number of other medical problems, some serious, some not. For example, any change in vision, hearing, tremors, unsteadiness of gait, and unexplained falls could indicate a tumor or a neurological disorder. If you have any of these symptoms, see your doctor, but do not assume the worst. The odds are in your favor.

Q. *I am pregnant and suffer from terrible migraines. My doctor advised me not to take any medication because it could pass through the placenta to the baby. Is there anything I can do about the pain?*

A. About 75 percent of all women with migraines will experience a worsening of their symptoms during pregnancy. Since many medications taken by the mother can pass through the placenta to the fetus and may cause birth defects, doctors are typically very cautious about allowing their patients to use painkillers. In these Situations, we need to carefully weigh the needs of the mother versus any potential risk to the baby. During the early stages of pregnancy, when the fetus is most likely to develop birth defects, pregnant women are advised not to use any medication stronger than acetaminophen, which is safe if taken in recommended doses. As any migraine sufferer knows, acetaminophen may barely make a dent in the headache, but it is certainly worth a try. If you can bear it, simply lie down and use an ice pack. If you are so sick that you cannot eat and are at risk of becoming dehydrated, which could harm both you and the baby, you must alert your doctor. In this situation, your physician may prescribe intravenous fluids and medication that will not harm your baby.

Although we do not want any woman to suffer unbearable pain, we are extremely cautious about the drugs we prescribe during pregnancy for good reason. Drug trials never include pregnant women intentionally, and because we have no good animal model of pregnancy that would allow us to test the effect of drugs on the developing fetus, we have no systematic way to test the consequences of giving any medication to a pregnant patient. Virtually all of our information comes from observing what has happened to the babies of women who have taken medication during pregnancy: that's how we learned thalidomide led to specific birth defects, for example—well after the fact!

Here's what we do know: Although some drugs that treat medical conditions cross the placenta, not all adversely affect the fetus, but some do and they must be discontinued. Lithium, which is a very effective medication for manic depressive illness, is teratogenic (causes malformations in the developing fetus), and patients on this medication must discontinue it during pregnancy. In general, the following guidelines are what physicians who take care of pregnant women try to follow:

- use no new drugs on the pregnant patient
- consult the medical literature for reports of fetal abnormalities in women taking established medications
- some chronic illnesses must be treated during pregnancy: hypertension and asthma are two good examples. In treating the pregnant woman with high blood pressure, it is usually safe to continue her medications with one exception: The class of drugs called angiotensin-converting enzyme inhibitors (ACE inhibitors) like Vasotec (enalapril) should not

be used and another category of medication has to be substituted. The drugs we use to control asthma (theophylline, beta-two agonist bronchodilators, and even steroids for managing acute and severe episodes of asthma) are all safe during pregnancy. Some, like theophylline, might be metabolized a little differently in the pregnant patient, so drug levels should be monitored carefully.

Heart

Q. *Does menopause increase a woman's risk of having a heart attack? What does estrogen have to do with the heart; I thought it was a sex hormone?*

A. Women have a lower risk of heart disease than men until they reach menopause, when, with each passing year, the risk of having a heart attack or being stricken with some other cardiovascular ailment increases. There is some controversy as to whether this increase is actually due to menopause or is merely a result of aging. In fact, diseases of the heart and blood vessels are the number-one killer of both men and women, and are responsible for the deaths of 500,000 women annually.

Until the past few years, we really did not know what, if anything, protected premenopausal women from heart disease. Several theories abounded, many of them were downright unscientific. For example, some researchers speculated that since men went to work and women typically stayed home raising children, women somehow had "easier" lives than men, which gave them protection against heart disease, at least in their younger years. (Whoever conjured up this theory has obviously never spent any time at home caring for children and running a household!) Other researchers

128

speculated that it was a protective effect of estrogen and that the hormone must offer some cardiovascular benefits that are lost after menopause, but no one ever examined what these benefits might be. It is only recently that scientists have begun to examine the particular role estrogen may play in warding off heart disease.

In recent years, there have been several fascinating findings about estrogen that have helped to shed light on the role this hormone plays in the cardiovascular system. What is particularly interesting is that estrogen appears to offer protection in many different ways, on many different fronts. Here is a review of some of the main findings:

- Prevents oxidative damage: Estrogen is an antioxidant.
- Improves blood lipids: When given to postmenopausal women in the form of HRT, estrogen raises high-density lipoproteins (HDLs or "good cholesterol") and lowers low-density lipoproteins (LDLs or "bad cholesterol"). LDL is the body's main carrier of cholesterol. Although cholesterol is essential for many body functions, too much causes cardiovascular disease. Excess cholesterol may be converted into plaque, a waxy substance that can clog the arteries delivering blood to the heart and other vital organs. On the other hand, HDL carries excess cholesterol out of the bloodstream so it can be excreted by the body. What is the right amount of LDL and HDL? Women should have an HDL value of 45 mg./dl. or above; ideally, LDL levels should be below 130 mg./dl.
- Improves blood flow: Women in particular are prone to constriction of the coronary arteries. This happens when the muscle cells in the arterial wall contract and narrow the diameter of the artery. Arteries may even go into prolonged spasm, thus preventing an adequate flow of blood to the heart muscle. In several studies, estrogen has been shown to prevent the constriction of the coronary arteries in women (although not in men). For example, in one study performed in London, researchers measured the diameter of the coronary arteries and the amount, of blood flowing through them, of nine postmenopausal women and seven men. They remeasured blood flow after introducing estrogen and a natural substance (acetylcholine) that causes constriction of diseased arteries. The researchers first injected the arteries with acetylcholine, and then injected estrogen. At first the arteries constricted, but within twenty minutes after the infusion of estrogen, the arteries relaxed, and coronary flow normalized in the women.

Clearly, estrogen, both naturally produced within the body and when taken orally, offers some excellent protection against heart disease. The more we learn about estrogen, the more multifaceted its role in the body appears to be.

Q. *My husband's doctor told him to take a baby aspirin every other day to protect against heart disease. On the other hand, my doctor never said anything to me about taking aspirin. Is aspirin helpful to women, too?*

A. When Carol and I first wrote the *Female Heart* (published in 1992), aspirin was being touted as a hot new way to prevent heart disease, but we advised our readers that since women had not been included in any of the studies on aspirin, there was no way of knowing whether it would work as well for them. Since that time, new studies suggest that aspirin may indeed be a useful tool in helping to prevent heart disease for both men and women. Here's why. Aspirin is a blood thinner—that is, it prevents the clumping together of blood platelets, which is a first step for clot formation. If a clot lodges in the arteries bringing blood to the heart or the brain, it can cause a heart attack or stroke.

The Nurses' Health Study, which followed the health and lifestyle of more than 87,500 women over several decades, clearly showed the beneficial effect of aspirin in moderate doses. In this study, those women who took one to six aspirin per week had a 30 percent reduction in the risk of first heart attack. These women were not taking aspirin to prevent heart disease, but were using it to treat other problems such as headaches or arthritis. The study also suggested that too much aspirin can be harmful; women who took more than seven aspirin per week did not show a reduction in the risk of first heart attack. This could also mean, however, that these women were simply sicker to begin with, and needed more aspirin to treat their various ailments.

The problem with the Nurse's Study is that it relies heavily on the accurate reporting of the participants themselves and, therefore, is not as valid as a more controlled study in which the information is gathered in a more objective way. A better and more extensive study on the effect of aspirin on postmenopausal women is currently under way. The Nurse's Health Study is a randomized, double-blind, placebo-controlled trial among more than 40,000 postmenopausal female nurses. This trial will test the risks and benefits of giving women 100 mg. of aspirin every other day. The results of this study should answer many of our questions about aspirin and women.

(Aspirin does not only offer protection against heart disease, it may also help to prevent colon cancer. A study of more than 635,000 men and women conducted by the American Cancer Society showed that those who took aspirin were at a significantly reduced risk of dying from cancers of the digestive tract.)

Many doctors are already convinced that aspirin is good protection against heart disease, and are recommending it for their patients. To protect against heart disease, the usual dose of aspirin is one baby aspirin every other day for both men and women.

As effective as aspirin may be, it may not be good for everyone. Even in small doses, aspirin can be irritating to the stomach lining and cause bleeding and ulcers in some people. Women who are taking aspirin should be closely monitored by their physicians for signs of gastrointestinal distress.

Q. *Is there any evidence that antioxidants can protect women against heart disease?*

A. Antioxidants are substances that prevent cells from being damaged by free radicals, which are unstable molecules that can cause malignant changes in cells. Damage to blood lipids by free radicals are believed to set in motion the process that causes the formation of plaque, the deposits of fat and cholesterol in the arteries that can cause atherosclerosis and can lead to heart attack. Several studies have strongly suggested that antioxidants may protect against heart disease, although many of these studies did not include women. One study however, did, (the Nurses's Health Study), and showed a positive link between the intake of two well-known antioxidants, vitamin E and beta-carotene, and a reduced risk of heart disease. In this study, the women who reported the highest intake of vitamin E, either through diet or supplements, had a 44 percent lower risk of heart disease than women with the lowest intake. Women with the highest intake of beta-carotene had a 22 percent reduction in the risk of coronary heart disease than women with the lowest intake. This study is hardly definitive, but it does add to the growing body of evidence that shows that antioxidants may reduce the risk of heart disease.

Q. *My mother, who is seventy-five, has a cholesterol level of 240. I am forty-eight, and my cholesterol level is 230. We go to the same doctor. At my last physical, my doctor advised me to reduce my cholesterol, and suggested changing my diet, and if necessary taking medication to bring it down. When my mother went in for her checkup, however, he said that her cholesterol was fine. Why the double standard?*

A. When it comes to cholesterol levels and the risk of heart disease, the rules change based on the age of the patient:

- In women fifty and under, the higher the levels of serum cholesterol, the greater the risk of heart disease.
- At all ages, women's HDL ("good cholesterol") level should be above 45.

- After age seventy, however, there is a weak correlation between cholesterol levels and the incidence of heart disease. At this age, we do not recommend lowering cholesterol through either drugs or diet unless values are over 260 mg./dl.

With the exception of people over seventy, cholesterol levels over 200 are a major risk factor for coronary artery disease in men. Frankly, we do not have enough data yet on whether this is true for women. We do know, however, that lowering total cholesterol level as well as the level of LDL ("bad cholesterol") in women does slow the progress of coronary heart disease.

Q. *What is the best way for a postmenopausal woman to lower a high cholesterol count and to raise her HDLs?*

A.There are several ways for a woman to lower her total serum cholesterol levels and to raise her HDLs. You can pop a pill that will slash your cholesterol or you can first try to make some constructive changes in your lifestyle, and use medication only as a last resort. The mode of treatment largely depends on the seriousness of the problem (in some cases, if a cholesterol is dangerously high, a physician may go straight for the medication) and the patient's willingness and ability to do what is necessary. Here are some of your options:

Diet Cutting back on fat, particularly saturated fat, is essential for lowering cholesterol levels. Saturated fat is found primarily in meat and whole-fat dairy products (milk, cheese, sour cream, ice cream) and is converted into cholesterol in the body. If you are eating a typical American diet, which is relatively high in saturated fat, reducing your intake of saturated fat is often all it takes to bring down total cholesterol. In order to do this effectively, you need to restrict your intake of saturated fat to under 10 percent of your total daily calories. I recommend asking your doctor for a referral to a qualified nutritionist who can help you devise an appropriate diet. There are also several excellent books on the subject, including *Dr. Dean Ornish's Program for Reversing Heart Disease* (Random House, 1990) and *Dean Ornish's Eat More, Weigh Less* (HarperCollins, 1993).

Women who diet must couple their changed eating habits with vigorous exercise because when women simply diet, they also lower their HDL's.

Exercise Exercise is a particularly effective way for a postmenopausal woman to raise her HDLs and lower her LDLs. In fact, studies have shown that when a sedentary woman embarks on a vigorous exercise program, her

132

HDL levels rise progressively as her exercise levels increase. Walking, running, jogging, cycling are some examples of "heart healthy" exercises. Whatever you do, it needs to be done on a regular basis—at least four times a week for forty-five minutes. If you work with an exercise trainer, I would recommend that your trainer at least initially talk with your doctor to plan the program that is best for you. (If you are over thirty-five or have been sedentary, do not start any exercise program without consulting your doctor.)

Estrogen There are several drugs that are given to both men and women to reduce cholesterol, and although they are effective, many people experience some undesirable side effects, notably gastrointestinal distress. The National Cholesterol Education Panel (NCEP), the group of medical professionals who devise national guidelines, recommends that before a woman is put on a lipid-altering drug, estrogen replacement therapy should first be considered. As I wrote earlier, estrogen has been shown to have a positive effect on blood lipids (it lowers total cholesterol, lowers LDLs, and raises HDLs); however, some women may not be good candidates for estrogen, or the estrogen therapy may not reduce their cholesterol enough. These women may have to take drugs that are specifically designed to reduce cholesterol.

Cholesterol busters Some of my women patients have normal or even below normal levels of total cholesterol but dangerously low HDL levels (below 35). The only option I can offer such women if exercise and estrogen replacement don't raise their HDL levels is to lower total cholesterol until the cholesterol/HDL level is lower than 4.4. If a woman has a dangerously high cholesterol, even when her HDL is normal or above 60 mg./dl. (which NCEP says is a positive protection for women from coronary artery disease), I then recommend one of the cholesterol-lowering drugs. I only do this when I have exhausted all other possibilities and it is absolutely necessary for my patient's health and well-being. Unfortunately, there have been very few studies to show whether these drugs are as effective in women as they are in men. Recently, however, a groundbreaking study in the journal *Circulation*, published by the American Heart Association, showed that at least one of these drugs worked well in women. In this study, sixty-two women who had atherosclerosis were given either lovastatin (sold as Mevacor) or a placebo. After sixteen weeks of treatment, the women taking lovastatin showed a dramatic 24 percent decrease in total cholesterol and a 32 percent drop in LDL ("bad" cholesterol"). (Both measurements went down by only 3 percent or less for the women on the placebo.) What was even more remarkable was that during follow-up examinations two years later, the majority of women taking lovastatin did not show any further narrowing of their coronary arteries, which

133

showed that the lovastatin had dramatically slowed down the destructive effect of atherosclerosis. On the other hand, the majority of the women on the placebo showed significant narrowing of the coronary arteries, a sign that their disease was progressing rapidly.

Although cholesterol-lowering drugs can be true lifesavers, these drugs can also have some unpleasant side effects, including constipation, nausea, headache, fatigue, and other annoyances. Some of these drugs can also cause more serious problems such as cataracts, gallstones, muscle destruction, and liver problems. If you are taking any of these drugs, you need to be closely monitored by your doctor.

Q. *My friends tell me that I am too tightly wound and if I don't learn how to relax I am going to have a heart attack. Are they right? Is there such a thing as a heart attack—prone personality?*

A. Although stress is not officially recognized as a bona fide risk factor for heart disease, there is a growing acknowledgment among physicians of the role stress may play in the disease process in general and in the progression of heart disease in particular.

Stress is not just experienced by the brain; its effects are keenly felt by nearly every cell in the body. Our body's response to stress is regulated by the autonomic or involuntary nervous system, which controls automatic functions such as blood pressure, breathing, and the beating of our hearts. The immediate response to stress is often called the "fight or flight" response—a defense mechanism scientists believe originated millions of years ago to help our ancestors cope with the dangers of primitive life. When we are confronted with a stressful situation, our bodies receive a message from our brains to gear up for action. The adrenal glands (located on top of the kidneys) begin to pump higher quantities of two hormones, epinephrine and norepinephrine, which, in turn, prepare the body for a burst of physical activity. The blood flow is directed away from the stomach to the skeletal muscles so that we can run faster; the kidneys begin to retain water and salt, which raises blood pressure so that the heart can pump more blood throughout the body. In the time of the cavemen, when the ability to outrun a rampaging animal could mean the difference between life and death, the fight or flight response was a true lifesaver. If stress is prolonged, another response kicks in, again due to the contribution of the adrenal glands, which make increased amounts of cortisone, a stress hormone. Scientists describe the response to chronic stress as "hypervigilance."

Today, stress is no longer a matter of avoiding a predator or hiding from a rival tribe. To the modern woman, stress is making sure the children are fed and dressed and their lunches packed before sending them off to school so that she can race to work. Stress is caring for ill parents, negotiating with intransigent bosses, calming irate clients, and worrying about paying the mortgage. Our bodies do not distinguish one kind of stress from another; when our brains detect stress, we experience the same physiological reactions as our ancestors, but the stress hormones are not used up in a burst of physical activity. They linger in the bloodstream slowly doing their damage. Over time, this kind of stress can be fatal.

Animal studies have shown that unrelenting stress can destroy otherwise healthy heart muscle. To minimize the effect of stress on either man or beast can be a deadly mistake. As biologist Robert M. Sapolsky notes in his fascinating book *Why Zebras Don't Get Ulcers,* after the SCUD missile attacks during the 1991 Persian Gulf War, more elderly Israelis suffered sudden cardiac death than those who were actually killed by the missiles themselves! In sum, stress can kill as swiftly and with greater destruction than even the most high-tech weapon.

Given all that we do know about stress, it is reasonable to assume that someone who is "tightly wound" or under a great deal of stress may indeed be at a somewhat higher risk of developing heart disease, especially in the presence of other risk factors. Not everyone who is under stress—even acute stress—will develop heart disease. The challenge is to identify the person who is particularly vulnerable and to intervene as early as possible. Through the years, there have been several studies that have attempted to identify the kind of personality that is more likely to fall prey to heart disease and the kinds of situations most likely to trigger it. As usual, the original research was done entirely of men, as were most other medical studies. In the 1970s, two famous researchers, Meyer Friedman, M.D., and Ray H. Rosenman, M.D., first coined the phrase Type A personality to describe the kind of aggressive, go-getting man who is most likely to end up in a cardiac care unit. Type A was a driven workaholic who demanded as much of himself as he did of others. The Type A man became the prototype of the heart attack personality until the 1980s, when a group at the National Institute of Aging introduced the concept of the "hostile personality" as a predictor for heart disease. Based on their studies, the man mostly likely to have a heart attack was not necessarily overworked or overly ambitious but arrogant, rude, argumentative, and surly. Little was known about the heart attack-prone women until the results of the famous Framingham Study, one of the first to include women subjects. The Framingham Study began in 1948 and followed the lives of men and women living in a small New England town. According to this study, the woman at greatest risk of having a heart attack is neither a Type A nor hostile personality: She is a passive woman who is married to a demanding or hostile Type A male. On the surface, this may seem puzzling. Why would a seemingly easy-going woman be a likely candidate for a heart attack? The answer has to do with the different ways men and women show anger, or, to be more precise, how men show anger and women don't. There is a whole body of literature that documents that from earliest childhood, girls are taught to be considerate of the feelings of others and to avoid confrontation at all costs, whereas boys are taught to ask directly for what they want. This is not necessarily all bad; being able to cajole a colleague or defuse a tense situation is a wonderful skill, up to a point. It is not, however, a skill that you want to practice twenty-four hours a day. Women who are in a position where they must continually placate difficult and demanding husbands, lovers, or children are under the worst kind of stress, and unlike the man who lashes out, they are taught to turn their anger, hostility, and frustration inward. It is these women whom I worry about the most and, ironically, are the least likely to ask for help.

Here are a couple of the things I recommend to patients to believe are under a great deal of stress.

Verbalize what the problem(s) actually is (are). This takes time, thought, and concentration. Begin by sitting clown quietly and write out what you believe your most serious problems actually are. Once you have done this, under each description, make two columns; list what is good about the problem (a difficult marriage might have some advantages, for example) and in the other column what is bad. Then read over the list of "bad" features and draw a line through what you believe you should or can no longer tolerate (for example, a husband's indifference may be bearable if he provides lavish financial support, but if he beats his wife, no compensation is enough reason to stay in the marriage).

Decide on a plan to escape from the troubling situation or problem in advance. This may require elaborate strategies and appropriate counseling. Credit card debt that seems insoluble might be best negotiated with the help of a debt counseling service. Escape from a troubling or painful relationship requires that you have a place to which you can go at least for an interim period until you are able to cope on your own. Once your plan is in place and as well worked out as possible, try to negotiate a solution with the other people involved. Make your statements simple and to the point; don't waste time on recrimination, shouting, or emotional scenes. You will discover that having your plan in place will make you able to negotiate your points much more effectively. State clearly what you can do and what you cannot—or will no longer—do. If the situation doesn't improve, try again to make your points clearly. A second failure to improve means it's time for you to put your escape plan into action.

The kind of sustained misery that produces heart attacks is always the same: It consists of a dilemma or a series of painful problems from which the sufferer feels she cannot escape and from which there seem to be no solutions. Some painful events, of course, are simply insoluble. The death of a beloved child or the loss of a home are blows that can't be reversed and simply have to be endured. For such tragedies, I advise the following:

- Change your environment if it's at all possible. Staying in the place where you lived with a loved person who has died is extremely painful.At least try to empty the room they occupied and change the decor. Try to put it to an entirely new use. Make a bedroom into a study or music room.
- Get enough sleep. If necessary, ask your doctor to prescribe a medication to help you get the rest you need. Exhaustion makes depression deepen.
- Eat nourishing food, even) in small portions. Take supplements if a loss of appetite continues to the point where you are losing weight and even hair. Your doctor can be very helpful in advising you as to which vitamins and food supplements might be most helpful.
- Exercise, exercise, exercise. Nobody playing a vigorous game of tennis can weep. Exercise raises the concentration of endorphins in the brain, relieves anxiety, and promotes both sleep and improved appetite.
- Get counseling if your grief or sense of stress doesn't relent. Even a wise, devoted friend might be helpful. Psychiatric attention can be lifesaving even if it's only necessary for a brief period of time.

Q. *I read that being depressed can increase the risk of having a heart attack. Is this true?*

A. Although we do not know why, a handful of studies have shown that a severe depression often precedes a heart attack, and it is particularly true in the case of second heart attacks. According to one recent Canadian study of 222 men and women who had already suffered heart attacks, those who had the most symptoms of depression (such as feeling sad, hopeless, unable to concentrate) were most likely to die of a second heart attack within eighteen months of their first. The researchers noted that the deaths among the depressed individuals were primarily due to irregular heartbeats called premature ventricular contractions. This is particularly interesting because we know that people under extreme stress or who are depressed often have hormonal imbalances that may upset the sympathetic nervous system, the body's automatic system that regulates such involuntary activities as blood pressure and heart rate. If the sympathetic nervous system is thrown out of whack, it

137

is very possible that it could cause disturbances in heart function. It may be possible that treating the depression may avert a second or even a first heart attack in susceptible people. This is not to say that every depressed person is going to have a heart attack, but if a person who is at high risk of heart disease shows signs of depression, it is advisable to seek both psychiatric and medical intervention.

There are many things about the body and the mind, and how the two are connected, that we simply do not yet fully understand. It is studies such as this one that confirm my belief that it is not enough for a doctor to simply check the patient's vital statistics; a doctor must be acutely aware of the subtle interactions between the physical and the emotional selves.

Q. I was recently diagnosed with mitral valve prolapse and I suffer from frequent and annoying heart palpitations. My doctor said that this condition was pretty common among women, and that there was nothing to worry about. Is there anything else I should know?

A. The mitral valve guards the opening between the atrium, the left upper chamber of the heart, and the ventricle, the left lower chamber. A mitral valve prolapse (MVP) is a developmental defect in which the leaflet of this valve becomes large, irregular in shape, and does not close as effectively as it should. As a result, some blood may leak back into the upper chamber when the heart contracts to pump blood forward to the rest of the body. MVP is usually not very serious and many people with this defect have absolutely no symptoms. About half of all MVP patients do complain of heart palpitations, skipped beats, or occasional chest pain. MVP is often detected upon physical examination when the physician hears through the stethoscope the telltale click and murmur that is typical of this condition. The diagnosis can be confirmed with an echocardiogram, a noninvasive test that provides a picture of the heart by producing and picking up sound waves reflected from the heart itself.

MVP affects about 6 percent of all women (and only 3 percent of men) and it tends to run in families. In a very small percent of cases, the MVP is so severe that the valve must be replaced with an artificial one.

Another small group of patients with MVP suffer from arrhythmias, which may be quite annoying, and heightened anxiety due to a hormonal imbalance in the sympathetic or involuntary nervous system. Often, these patients are successfully treated with a class of drugs called beta-blockers.

Most people with MVP can live perfectly normal, healthy lives and do not need to give much thought to this problem, with one exception: All MVP patients should take antibiotics before any procedure that will introduce bacteria into their bloodstream, such as a visit to the dentist and before childbirth or any kind of surgery. Many patients who are nauseated by the high doses of antibiotics they may need before their procedures may be tempted to skip them. Don't! There is a real albeit small possibility that the valves could become infected. Such an infection, subacute bacterial endocarditis, is difficult to cure and requires intravenous antibiotics over a period of weeks. In some cases, the infected valve may even have to be replaced. None of this need ever happen: It can be prevented simply by taking antibiotics prophylactically.

Q. *Sometimes, for no apparent reason, my heart starts to pound rapidly and then it stops. My friend told me that it was a sign of stress, but I'm worrying that I have a heart problem. Do I have anything to worry about?*

A. A rapid heartbeat could be a sign of stress but not necessarily. The normal heart beats about seventy times per minute and, in most cases, you are not even aware of it happening. There are a few situations in which it is quite normal to feel your heart beating or even racing in your chest—for example, when you're exercising, very nervous, or exerting yourself in some way. Some people may become aware of their heartbeat at night when they're lying down, particularly if they are lying on their left side. This is also normal and is nothing to worry about.

The feeling that your heart is skipping a beat, or that there is a sensation of "flipping" in your chest, occurs when there is one or more heartbeats from a site other than the usual pacemaker of the heart's rhythms. If you are feeling only a few early or extra beats (two or three), it is probably not serious, even if it happens frequently throughout the day. If, on the other hand, your heart has periods of very rapid beating (over 130 beats per minute) you need to consult your physician.

A rapid or irregular heartbeat could be an indication of a heart problem, but it could also be caused by many different physical and emotional problems, ranging from a high fever, anemia, an overactive thyroid gland, or excessive stress. Rapid heartbeat could also be caused by something as simple as too much caffeine (I have seen this in patients who survive on coffee and cola), a side effect of a medication, or a reaction to alcohol (especially hard liquor). Any patient with this problem should be thoroughly examined by her physician. Be prepared to tell the doctor when these rapid heart rates occur (at night, after exercise, at work?), how long they usually last, and whether there is any particular situation that seems to trigger them. Obviously, the treatment will depend on the diagnosis.

High Blood Pressure

Q. During my last physical, my doctor told me that I had high blood pressure and pre-scribed medication that she told me I would probably have to take for the rest of my life. In addition, she urged me to stop taking birth control pills. Frankly, I was shocked to hear that I had any problem at all. I felt very well and had lots of energy, at least until I started tak-ing the medicine. After a few days on the drug I felt tired and depressed, so I discontinued it. Now I feel fine again. Why should I continue to take medication that is making me feel worse than the actual problem? Is there anything else that I can do to control my blood pressure? Do I really have to stop taking birth control pills?

A. High blood pressure (also called hypertension) is one of the most difficult conditions to explain to patients because, in most cases, the patient feels fine. That is what is so deceptive about this insidious disease. High blood pressure does its damage quietly long before any symptoms develop. Suddenly, out of the blue, a patient who considers herself to be perfectly healthy is told that she must take medicine, not just for a few weeks but for an entire lifetime. What is even worse is that often the medicine, at least initially, causes unpleasant side effects. Most patients, like yourself, find this very bewilder-ing, and simply choose to ignore the diagnosis.

This could be the mistake of their lives. In order to understand why treatment for high blood pressure is so important, you need to understand the potential hazards of this condition.

When the heart pumps, it pushes blood through larger arteries into smaller ones called arterioles. When your doctor takes your blood pressure, she is measuring the force the blood exerts against the walls of the body's large arteries. The arterioles control the flow of blood throughout the body by either expanding or contracting. In the case of high blood pressure, the arterioles contract, thus reducing the total capacity of the vascular space into which the heart must eject its bolus of blood. As a result, the heart has to pump harder to maintain a normal blood flow throughout the body, and thus can become overworked and enlarged. If it is untreated, hypertension can have deadly consequences. High blood pressure scars and stiffens the walls of blood vessels, and injured arteries are more likely to accumulate plaque, deposits of fat, cholesterol, and other debris that can clog the vessels, restricting the flow of blood. In fact, high blood pressure is a leading cause of heart attack, stroke, kidney failure, and atherosclerosis (the narrowing of the arteries delivering blood to the heart).

In 90 to 95 percent of all cases of high blood pressure, the cause is unknown. In a small number of cases, high blood pressure is caused by a physical problem, such as a kidney abnormality, which can be corrected. Five percent of women on birth control pills will develop high blood pressure, and only half of the women who get high blood pressure on the Pill will return to normal levels when they stop taking it.

Blood pressure is measured by a sphygmomanometer or pressure gauge, a rubber cuff containing a bladder (an empty rubber sac) that is wrapped tightly around a person's arm over one of the large arteries. When the cuff is inflated, it compresses the artery in the arm, briefly stopping the flow of blood. The air in the cuff is then slowly released, and the physician (or medical technician) measuring the blood pressure listens with a stethoscope. When the blood begins to flow back through the artery, the pulsations of the blood through the vessel make a sound that can actually be heard. The pressure at which this occurs is called the systolic pressure and is the first number the doctor records. As the pressure in the cuff decreases, the sound disappears. When this happens, the pressure in the artery has exceeded that in the cuff. This value is the diastolic pressure, the second number the doctor records.

For a premenopausal woman, normal blood pressure is defined as anywhere between 110/65 and 120/80 mm/Hg (millimeters of mercury). High blood pressure is any measure over 140/90. Women tend to have lower blood pressure than men until after menopause, when the risk of developing high blood pressure is equal to that of men. Half of all women between the ages of fifty-five and sixty-four have high blood pressure, and more than two thirds of all women past sixty-five have high blood pressure. High blood pressure is a particularly devastating problem among African-American women, as underscored by the fact that 82 percent or more African-American women will die of strokes than white women.

It is not uncommon for the initial blood pressure reading be elevated. If your first value is high, your doctor will check it again in about ten minutes, when you are more relaxed. If your readings continue to be high, your doctor will talk to you about treatment options. Although we used to dismiss an initial high reading as so-called white-coat hypertension—in other words, it was unimportant because you were nervous about being examined—we now believe that it may be significant in that it shows that you may respond to stress in negative and unhealthy ways. Even if the second reading is lower, many doctors, myself included, will at the very least recommend a stress-control program, coupled with an exercise program, and, if necessary, weight loss.

Treatment for high blood pressure can include changes in lifestyle and, when necessary, medication.

Weight control Obesity increases the risk of high blood pressure. People who lose even just a few pounds almost always drop a few points off their blood pressure readings.

Diet Simple changes in diet may have a profound impact on blood pressure. It is important to monitor how much alcohol patients are drinking and whether or not they are consuming large quantities of caffeine. For some patients, lowering dietary salt may be sufficient. The American Heart Association recommends eating no more than 2 to 2.5 grams of sodium daily. In order to achieve this level, you must avoid processed foods and pass on the salt shaker.

Eating a diet high in fiber may also help to maintain normal blood pressure. According to a study conducted at the Harvard Medical School of more than 30,000 men, those who ate less than 12 grams of fiber per day were 60 percent more likely to develop high blood pressure over a four-year period. We don't know yet whether the same would be true for women, but a high-fiber diet has significant advantages for women, so it's worth trying.

Calcium, a mineral found in dairy products and green leafy vegetables, has also been shown to reduce the risk of high blood pressure. Try eating more yogurt, broccoli, kale, canned salmon or sardines with bones, and calcium-fortified fruit juice.

142

Exercise Regular exercise helps lower blood pressure and decreases stress. When we are under stress, our bodies produce chemicals that can raise blood pressure and rev our bodies up for action—the so-called fight or flight hormones. If we sit and simmer, these hormones linger in the bloodstream and keep our blood pressure at higher than normal levels. If we put these hormones to good use—that is, if we exercise—the blood pressure will return to normal faster. Riding a stationary bicycle for thirty minutes or walking two miles four times a week may be all it takes to control stress and reduce a high blood pressure reading. Check with your doctor before starting an exercise program to make sure your heart can handle the increased activity.

What other medication are you taking? Many over-the-counter products, particularly for allergies and colds, contain ephedrine, which can raise blood pressure in susceptible people. If you have high blood pressure, you should not use any cold or allergy medication without checking with your doctor.

As I said earlier, birth control pills can raise blood pressure in some women. If you have been diagnosed with high blood pressure, you should find some other form of contraception.

Medication There are times when despite your best efforts to reduce your blood pressure on your own, medication is necessary. Your physician will prescribe one or a combination of several drugs. They may include:

- Diuretics: These "water pills" rid the body of excess salt and water, thus reducing blood volume. Commonly prescribed diuretics include Diuril and Lasix.
- Alpha- or beta-blockers: Known as sympathetic nerve inhibitors, these prevent the constriction of the small arteries that control blood pressure.
- ACE inhibitors and calcium channel blockers: These drugs lessen the degree to which the muscles in the blood vessel wall constrict so that the vessel dilates or expands, thus reducing blood pressure.
- Centrally active agents: Some drugs, like clonidine, work by having an effect on the brain itself.

Although these drugs are effective in reducing blood pressure, they can each cause unpleasant side effects in some individuals. These include headache, depression, excessive fatigue, troublesome cough, and impotence. Many of these problems will wear off within a few weeks of beginning the medication. If you suffer any side effects, your physician may be able to alter your dose or switch you to another drug. It can be very dangerous to discontinue your blood pressure medicine without first consulting your doctor.

143

Iron Supplements

Q. *Several years ago, when I was suffering from extreme fatigue, I was diagnosed as having iron deficiency anemia, and my doctor suggested that I take an iron supplement. (I have very heavy menstrual periods and since I am watching my cholesterol, I do not eat much meat.) I took the supplement for several months and then Stopped when I felt better, but every once in a while when I feel like I'm getting anemic again, I take iron pills on my own. Recently, I read an alarming report that stated that an excess of iron can cause heart disease. Should I throw out my iron pills? How else should I be treating my anemia?*

A. If you are truly suffering from iron deficiency anemia, you are not endangering yourself in any way by taking an iron supplement if it is prescribed by your physician. Iron deficiency anemia is a very common problem among menstruating women, especially those who have excessive menstrual flow. The symptoms of iron deficiency anemia include fatigue, inability to concentrate (girls with this problem often do not perform as well in school as they should), and sometimes shortness of breath after mild exertion. Although it may not be life-threatening, iron deficiency anemia can be a very unpleasant and uncomfortable ailment that can interfere with a woman's quality of life. It should definitely be treated. Iron deficiency anemia can be diagnosed with a simple blood test, and is usually easily cured with an iron supplement. Premenopausal women need about 18 mg. of iron daily; it is often difficult for women to get enough iron from their food, especially those who are dieting and are steering clear of red meat, which may have an abundance of fat and calories but is an excellent source of iron. (Dried fruits, legumes, and iron-fortified cereals are also good sources of this mineral.) The iron found in food is most easily absorbed by the body. Calcium and fiber can block absorption of the type of iron found in supplements, and should not be taken at the same time as an iron pill. Vitamin C can enhance the absorption of iron; therefore, I advise patients to drink a glass of orange or cranberry juice with their iron supplement. It is also best to take an iron supplement between, not during or after, meals. Time-released supplements work the best. Since iron can cause constipation, I also advise using a supplement that includes a stool softener.

If you are not iron deficient, however, taking additional iron could pose a potential health risk, especially after menopause. As you noted, there have been studies that suggest that an excess amount of iron stored in the body may increase the risk of developing heart disease. In one highly publicized Finnish study, researchers found that men with the highest blood concentrations of ferritin (iron) were the ones who were most likely to have heart attacks. The researchers speculated that too much iron in the blood can promote the formation of free radicals—unstable molecules that can injure the cells lining the artery walls and actually damage heart muscle. This was not a convincing study, by the way, and the mere finding of an association between high stores of iron and coronary artery disease does not prove the former caused the latter! The most characteristically nonsensical feature of the study was the extrapolation of the supposed conclusion to women: The authors suggested that women were protected from heart disease while menstruating because their iron stores were often low as a result of their reproductive cycling. I remember being asked to comment on the study while on a speaking tour and marveling at the time about how work done exclusively on men was extrapolated to women without a qualm.

Although iron deficiency anemia is not as common among menopausal women as it is in women who are still menstruating, it can and does occur among the elderly population. This is usually due to years of inadequate nutrition: I call it the "tea and toast" anemia. Many older people suffer from all or some causes of decreased pleasure in food (an impaired sense of smell that affects taste, medications that dry the mouth, depression, and poverty) and have very little interest in eating. They will often eat the same things every day, particularly if they find shopping for fresh foodstuffs difficult.

We know that a woman's risk of heart disease increases with increasing age. Until recently, most researchers believed the increased risk was solely due to the drop in estrogen production with menopause. Many scientists are now beginning to rethink this hypothesis and are wondering if iron may also play a role in heart disease. It makes sense that it may. A woman stops menstruating with menopause, which means she is no longer losing blood on a monthly basis, thus allowing iron stores to build up in her blood. If excessive iron does indeed promote the formation of free radicals, then it could very well be that too much iron could be at least one of the factors involved in the increased risk of heart disease after menopause. In fact, one Norwegian study of 113 premenopausal and 46 post-menopausal women confirmed that iron levels rise sharply after menstrual bleeding stops. The researchers found some other compelling facts: high iron levels also correlated positively with higher total cholesterol levels and in particular, higher levels of LDL ("bad cholesterol").

I do not advise any woman to take an iron supplement without first having a blood test to determine if she is iron deficient. Do not assume that fatigue and listlessness are necessarily signs of iron deficiency; there are other types of anemia that are due to a lack of certain B vitamins. Taking iron will not correct them. In addition, excessive tiredness could be a symptom of many different problems that can only be detected during a physical examination.

After menopause, the need for iron drops, and some researchers believe that the daily iron intake should drop to roughly half of what it was (to about 9 mg.). At this stage in life, women should be careful about controlling their iron intake, but this may not be as easy as it sounds. Even if you make it a point to cut back on red meat and other iron-rich foods, iron can still be found in many multivitamin supplements and in fortified foods such as cereals and bread. Learn to read labels for hidden sources of iron: I would not advise eating iron-fortified foods or taking a vitamin supplement with iron unless it is under the advice of your physician.

Medical Tests

Q. *I have just turned forty and have become concerned about my health. What medical tests should I have each year?*

A. There is no "official" list that clearly spells out which medical tests are required for all patients. In fact, the list of which tests should be given varies according to who is doing the recommending. For example, the American Heart Association advises people over forty to have an annual electrocardiogram (EKG), but other medical groups do not. Some medical groups urge women past forty to have annual mammograms, others say it is unnecessary until age fifty. Therefore, it is up to your doctor to decide which tests are appropriate for you. I personally feel that the annual physical examination for the average-risk female patient age forty and over should include the following:

- a blood pressure reading: Every woman should have her blood pressure checked annually. High blood pressure is known as the "silent killer" because it is painless and symptomless, yet it can be deadly. (For more information on blood pressure, see page 138.)
- a manual breast examination by a knowledgeable physician

147

- a mammogram every two years; annually after age fifty (For more information on mammograms, see page 50.)
- a fecal blood occult test: In this test, the physician takes a stool sample and sends it to a laboratory to test for hidden blood. Bleeding could be a sign of colon cancer. This test should be performed annually after age fifty.
- a digital rectal exam: In this test, the physician inserts a gloved finger into the rectum and feels for any growths, abnormalities, or signs of bleeding.
- a flexible sigmoidoscopy: In this examination, the physician inserts a soft fiberoptic tube into the rectum, providing a good view of the lower colon. If I detect a polyp or other problem, I would send my patient for a colonoscopy, which allows the physician to view the entire colon.
- serum blood lipid profile: Given the fact that heart disease is the number-one killer of women, I believe it is essential to monitor total cholesterol, HDL, LDL, and triglycerides, as well as fasting blood sugar to check for signs of glucose intolerance, a precursor to heart disease. (For a more complete explanation, see page 126.)
- a thyroid function test: In this test, a blood sample is taken and analyzed at a laboratory for levels of thyroid hormone.
- a bone density test: By age forty-five, I order a bone density test to check for osteoporosis, and to use as a baseline to determine future bone loss.
- a Pap smear (to check for cervical cancer) and a manual pelvic exam to check for any abnormalities
- an electrocardiogram (EKG): This painless, noninvasive test lets the physician see if the heart has sustained any damage due to oxygen deprivation (signs of a heart attack), or if there is an irregular heartbeat. Since more than one third of all heart attacks in women are "silent"that is, they go undetected—I feel this test is essential.
- serum estradiol level: Around the time of perimenopause (age forty-five or so), when estrogen levels begin to decline, I recommend that women have a simple blood test to check their serum estradiol levels at least every two years to determine if they require hormone replacement therapy.
- other tests for special situations: Depending on personal and family history, other medical tests may be ordered. For example, if a woman is at risk of glaucoma—an eye disease that can cause blindness if left untreated—she should be tested annually for this problem by her primary care physician or an ophthalmologist. If a patient complains about hearing loss, she should have her hearing checked and monitored annually. I often recommend that smokers have annual chest X-rays—I have picked up lung cancers twice this year on "routine" chest films. And if a patient has been sexually active but has not been practicing "safe sex," I would urge her to have a test for HIV or other sexually transmitted diseases.

Menopause

Q. *I am fifty-one years old and have begun showing signs of menopause. Half of my friends are on hormone replacement therapy and swear by it; the other half simply would not even consider taking hormones. I am so confused on this issue: How does a woman know which decision is right for her?*

A. The decision of whether to go on hormone replacement therapy—HRT (combination estrogen/progesterone therapy)—is not one that a woman should make alone or based on the experiences of her friends; it is an important medical decision that should be made in collaboration with her doctor. Every menopausal woman should be carefully evaluated by her doctor, and then presented with a clear picture of both the benefits—which are many—and the risks—which are real—of taking hormones. Once a woman knows the facts, as well as her personal risk factors, she and her physician can then decide what is best for her. Before taking hormone replacement therapy, here are some important facts that every woman should know.

Until recently (within the past two or three years) the prevailing opinion in much of the medical community was that every menopausal woman, with few exceptions, could benefit from taking hormones. HRT was touted as a veritable fountain of youth, a wonder drug that could not only keep you slim, sexy, and young, but could prevent heart disease and osteoporosis. There may be some doctors who still feel this way, but most realize the decision to recommend hormone replacement therapy for women must be made on an individual basis. The findings of the Nurse's Health Study, conducted by the Harvard Medical School, is one reason why some doctors are somewhat less than enthusiastic about hormones. This highly publicized study found that taking HBT for more than five years could increase a woman's risk of getting breast cancer. In fact, for women between the ages of fifty and sixty-four who had been on HRT for more than five years, breast cancer risk increased 40 percent over normal; for women between the ages of sixty-five and sixty-nine, the increase was 70 percent. What this means in real numbers is that a woman aged fifty to fifty-four on HRT for more than five years has a 1 in 320 chance of getting breast cancer, versus a 1 in 450 risk if she had taken HRT for fewer than five years, and a woman between the ages of sixty-five and sixty-nine who has been on HRT for five years has a 1 in 144 risk of getting breast cancer versus a 1 in 244 if she had been on HRT for fewer years.

Although statisticians will argue that the risk of developing breast cancer on HRT is still relatively small, it is nevertheless, something that doctors must consider before writing out a prescription. It is also important to note that many other studies have found absolutely no link between HRT and breast cancer, and many doctors, including oncologists, are skeptical that such a link exists, or if it does, whether it is significant. This does not mean that you can ignore the findings of the Nurse's Study, merely that you must carefully weigh the risk of breast cancer against the potential benefits of HRT.

Who is HRT for? There should be a compelling reason for a doctor to prescribe HRT—the fact that a woman is menopausal is not enough. The decision to prescribe estrogen should be made on the basis of one or more of the following situations:

Intolerable menopausal symptoms Some women can breeze through menopause without so much as a hot flash. Others, however, are not so lucky. Many are made truly miserable by common menopausal symptoms, such as insomnia or frequent night awakenings often due to hot flashes, depression, painful sexual intercourse due to the thinning of the vaginal walls, and frequent urinary tract infections, in addition, many women experience a marked change in cognitive ability—that is, they have difficulty concentrating and often show a loss in short-term memory. These normal symptoms of menopause can be lessened, if not completely cured, by taking HRT.

Osteoporosis Estrogen is involved in the absorption of calcium by the bones, which is critical for the formation of new bone. As estrogen levels dip after menopause, every woman experiences an acceleration in the rate at which she is losing bone. She may lose so much that she develops osteoporosis, a dangerous thinning of the bones which make them likely to fracture. Studies have shown that HRT can help stem the loss of bone mass and thus can prevent osteoporosis. At menopause, every woman should have a bone density test to determine her risk of developing osteoporosis. If the bone density test reveals a lower than normal bone density in the vertebral spine or hips (the areas that are most prone to breaks), she should consider taking HRT.

Coronary artery disease HRT has many positive effects on the heart. Among other things HRT can:

- Increase the level of HDL ("good cholesterol"), which protects against heart disease.
- Prevent the oxidation of LDL ("bad cholesterol"), which raises the risk of heart disease.
- Prevent the arteries from constricting or narrowing, thus helping to maintain the flow of blood to the heart and throughout the body.
- Reduces the stickiness of formed elements in the blood, thus lessening the possibility of an occluded artery.

Based on what we know about HRT, in the long run, hormone replacement therapy may prove to be a potent treatment against heart disease. Unfortunately, there have not been any long-term prospective, double-blind clinical studies examining this issue. The Nurse's Study did show that HRT users had a 40 percent reduction in risk of coronary artery disease compared with the general population. But critics of the study contend that it is not clear whether the HRT itself was responsible for this reduction or simply whether women who take hormones have a healthier lifestyle than women who don't. The reasoning is, if a woman is concerned about her health enough to take hormones, she may eat a more prudent diet, exercise more, visit her doctor more, and, in sum, take better care of herself. Even though it is not yet a proven fact, I feel that there is at least solid circumstantial evidence that HRT can have a beneficial effect on women with heart disease or at high risk of developing heart disease. Specifically, I recommend that HRT should be considered for women who have at least two risk factors for heart disease and an HDL below 35 mg./dl.

Who should avoid HRT? Generally, we do not recommend HRT for women who smoke, have a history of blood clots, have had breast cancer or are at high risk of getting breast cancer, or have a history of endometriosis or uterine cancer. We would also be wary about prescribing HRT to a woman with a history of migraine headaches, since estrogen can aggravate this condition, although this is not true for all women with migraines. In fact, some do fine on HRT. I would also be wary about prescribing HRT for women with a history of asthma. According to the Nurses' Health Study, women who reported using HRT at any time were 50 percent more likely to suffer from asthma than women who never took hormones. Women who took hormones for ten or more years had twice the normal incidence of asthma. Although severe childhood asthma is more common among boys than girls, in adults, more women than men suffer from serious forms of asthma. Researchers have long suspected a link between female hormones and asthma, but they do not yet understand the effect estrogen may have on the respiratory system.

I want to stress that when it comes to HRT, there really aren't any hard-and-fast rules. For example, if a woman who is cured of breast cancer develops heart disease, her physician may decide that the risk of her dying from a heart attack is much greater than a recurrence of cancer, and therefore put her on HRT. I have done this with the collaboration of a skilled breast surgeon, who with me monitors the patient very closely for a recurrence of malignancy. When a woman at high risk for developing breast cancer is so miserable because of her menopausal symptoms that she is unable to function, her physician may prescribe HRT for a short period to help her through this difficult time. Obviously, these patients would need to be monitored very closely.

What HRT may do Recent studies have shown that the benefits of estrogen may be more widespread than was ever imagined. Among other things, HRT has been linked to a lower rate of Alzheimer's disease, a significant reduction in the risk of colon cancer, and may even help to prevent degeneration, the most common form of blindness in the elderly. Estrogen also appears to have a cosmetic effect on the skin, helping to maintain skin thickness and moisture.

As good as HRT sounds, keep in mind that the use of hormones is relatively new—few women have taken hormones for more than a decade, and we simply do not know the long-term effects of this treatment. Although early studies have been quite promising, it will take years before we can say with any certainty that the long-term use of hormones is safe or that it is even effective. In the meantime, it is essential that HRT be given selectively to the patients who will most benefit from it.

Estrogen can be taken in several ways: The preparation we know most about is Premarin, a mixture of hormones of the estrogen family obtained from the urine of pregnant mares. There are also pure preparations of a single active estrogen, estradiol, which are taken in tablet form. Oral estrogen preparations are best taken in the morning after eating, and some experts recommend that estradiol pills be taken twice daily in a divided dose after meals so that there is no fall-off in blood estrogen concentrations as the day wears on. Estrogen administration should continue 365 days a year and, ideally, should not be interrupted. Women who complain of breast engorgement and pain, however, may do better if they have a few days a month without estrogen.

Estrogen can also be delivered by a group of transdermal preparations (patches) that are applied to a patch of hair-free skin; these are changed periodically. Estrogen is delivered in a steady supply to the bloodstream by this method and the drug does not have to be absorbed and processed by the liver, as happens with an oral preparation.

All women on estrogen replacement therapy who have not had hysterectomies *must* also take progestin, which prevents the buildup and malignant transformation of the cells lining the uterus. Progestins can be given daily in small doses; this will eliminate menstrual bleeding in most women within three or four months. Others may wish to cycle and these patients use progestins for only twelve days of their cycle. Progestins should be taken at night because they are vasoconstrictors (narrows the arteries) and may produce arterial narrowing, which, in susceptible women, may lead to a decreased blood supply to vital organs like the brain.

Estrogen-containing creams that are inserted directly into the vagina are useful for women who cannot tolerate or who do not wish to use full regimens of hormone replacement therapy. Properly used, these creams allow dry, atrophied vaginal linings to renew themselves, improving lubrication and often eliminating painful intercourse.

Q. *I've been on HRT for two years. When I visited my internist for my annual checkup, he asked me if I had been getting an annual endometrial biopsy. My gynecologist, who had prescribed the hormone therapy, had never mentioned this test to me. I do get an annual Pap smear, and have always believed that was enough to detect any gynecological problems. Do I need an endometrial biopsy also?*

A. Judging by how many questions I am asked on this particular issue, there appears to be a great deal of confusion about endometrial biopsies and hormone replacement therapy. Here are the facts: When postmenopausal hormone replacement therapy was first introduced more than two decades ago, estrogen was given alone, or, as we say, "unopposed" by other hormones. Although estrogen helped relieve many of the unpleasant symptoms of menopause, it had one undesirable and potentially dangerous side effect: It stimulated the build up of blood in the uterine lining (the endometrium), which increased the risk of uterine cancer. As a result, women who were taking estrogen were routinely given a test called an endometrial biopsy. In this test, the physician inserts a small catheter into the uterus via the vagina through a tiny opening in the cervix, the circular indentation at the mouth of the uterus. During this procedure, cells from the lining of the uterus, the endometrium, are sucked out through the catheter and later examined under a microscope for signs of cancerous changes. The patient may experience some cramping during or after the biopsy, but most patients do not need anything stronger for pain relief than an ibuprofen tablet.

An endometrial biopsy is a much more accurate and thorough test for uterine cancer than a Pap smear, in which cells are collected just from the cervix. Around ten years ago, however, pharmaceutical companies introduced the estrogen/progesterone pill, which greatly reduced the risk of uterine cancer. Progesterone is a hormone that causes the endometrial lining to shed, similar to a menstrual cycle, thus preventing the buildup of the endometrial lining and reducing the risk of uterine cancer. Today, most women are taking the estrogen/progesterone combination and, therefore, are not routinely given endometrial biopsies. A woman on combination therapy will be given a biopsy if she experiences any abnormal bleeding, which may be due to a cancer or other type of growth. If you are taking the combination pill and are not having any problems, your gynecologist is correct that you do not need an endometrial biopsy. If, however, you are taking pure estrogen, you should follow the advice of your internist and get an annual endometrial biopsy.

Q. *I have just become menopausal, and my gynecologist recommended that I take HRT I told him that I didn't want to take HRT because when I had been on the pill many years ago, I found that estrogen made me very moody. My doctor said that the estrogen used today is a much lower dose than in the past, and (this is an exact quote) "Every intelligent woman in my practice is taking hormones." Help! I don't want to take hormones. Are there any alternatives to HRT?*

A. First, let me reassure you that I know many intelligent women—I count myself among them—who for various reasons are not on hormone replacement therapy. Although there are many benefits to HRT, it is not for everyone. My advice is, find yourself a doctor who is more open-minded, and more willing to consider each patient's individual feelings and needs.

If one of my patients is unable or unwilling to take HRT, we work out an alternative program to maintain maximum health and fitness, depending on her needs:

Help for hot flashes and depression As a woman's body adjusts to the diminishing levels of estrogen, she may experience some unpleasant symptoms, such as hot flashes or mild depression. Many women report that vitamins C and E can help relieve hot flashes. I recommend my menopausal patients take 1,000 mg. of vitamin C and 800 units of vitamin E daily. Women who suffer from depression or moodiness, other common complaints of menopausal women, may be helped by taking 200 mg. of vitamin B6, which is reputed to be a natural mood enhancer. (Excess amounts of B6 can cause nerve damage, so do not exceed the recommended dose.)

Vaginal dryness Women who suffer from vaginal dryness can use topical estrogen-containing creams that can restore some of the tone and elasticity to the vaginal wall. Many women who are reluctant about taking hormones internally are more comfortable about using estrogen topically because little of the hormone is absorbed into the bloodstream. Women who want or need to avoid estrogen in any form can use non-hormonal vaginal moisturizing creams, which are sold over-the-counter in premeasured, disposable plastic applicators. They are inexpensive and easy to use. Vitamin E is also reputed to ease the vaginal dryness that can occur after menopause, although there are no studies that I am aware of that have proven or disproved this. Women who have reported good results with this vitamin have taken between 800 and 1200 units daily of vitamin E. (The Recommended Daily Allowance for vitamin E is 400 units. Women who are taking blood thinners should not use vitamin E.)

Heart protectors Estrogen has been shown to significantly reduce the risk of heart disease, the leading cause of death in women. Vitamins E, C, and A (beta-carotene) can retard the development of plaque in the arteries, which can lead to a heart attack. Once a woman reaches menopause, her risk of having a heart attack soars with each passing year. Many studies have shown that antioxidants can help maintain normal cholesterol levels, thus warding off heart disease. Vitamin B6 is also important for the prevention of heart disease. Recently, researchers found that a supplement of 200 mg. of vitamin B6 helped to maintain normal blood levels of a protein called homocysteine. Elevated levels of homocysteine have been linked to a dramatic increase in the risk of having a heart attack.

Weight control When estrogen levels drop, many women develop a tendency toward midline obesity; in other words, their waistlines disappear. If there is any weight gain, the weight will settle in the midline area, which is not only unattractive but, more important, can increase the risk of having a heart attack. It is essential, therefore, for women to maintain normal weight after menopause. Regular aerobic exercise can not only improve cardiovascular fitness but can burn extra calories.

The right amount of dietary fat HRT raises the level of HDLs, the so-called good cholesterol that protects against heart disease. The ratio of total cholesterol to HDL should be below 4.4. In women (but not in men), a low-fat diet can often result in a decrease in HDLs. Therefore, women who are dieting to lose weight should have their HDL levels measured on a regular basis. If their HDLs fall too low, they may need to add more fat to their diet. (I'm not talking about ingesting a huge amount of fat: a tablespoon or two of olive oil daily may do the trick.) Vigorous exercise on a regular basis can also raise HDL levels in women.

Osteoporosis Estrogen protects against osteoporosis, a debilitating bone disease that can cause brittle, thin bones that break easily. Complications from bone fractures are a leading cause of death among older women. If a woman is not taking HRT, she must be vigilant about finding other ways to protect herself against osteoporosis. I recommend that these women take a calcium supplement of 1,500 mg. daily along with 400 units of vitamin D. A good exercise program consisting of 30-40 minutes a day of weight-bearing exercise, such as lifting weights or walking briskly, can help retain bone mass.

Q. *When I go to my health food store, I see row upon row of pills and potions designed to help ease the symptoms of menopause. Are these products safe? Can you recommend any in particular?*

A. Like that of most physicians, my medical training did not include any courses on alternative medicine; therefore, I cannot answer your question with any real authority. I did ask Fredi Kronenberg, M.D., the director of the Richard and Hinda Rosenthal Center for Complementary and Alternative Medicine at the College of Physicians and Surgeons at Columbia University, whether she could recommend any natural treatments for menopause. Unfortunately, Dr. Kronenberg said, none of these products have yet undergone any well-controlled scientific clinical studies to determine their safety and efficacy. This is not to say that they are unsafe or that they don't work; we simply don't know. Studies are currently being planned, but so far there is no concrete evidence.

Although I don't recommend it to my patients, some women in my practice swear that ginseng, a popular supplement, has helped relieve many of the symptoms of menopause. For thousands of years, Chinese healers have used ginseng to treat "women's problems." There are no clinical studies to back up this claim; however, we do know that ginseng contains compounds called phytoestrogens, hormonelike substances that mimic the action of estrogen in humans. Many plant foods, in particular soybeans, contain high levels of phytoestrogens. The Japanese in particular eat a great deal of foods made from soy, notably tofu. Studies have shown that Japanese women do not appear to experience hot flashes or many of the other unpleasant symptoms of menopause typical among Western women. In fact, recently, the *New England Journal of Medicine* published a letter from Dr. Herman Aldercreutz, a leading researcher in the field of phytoestrogens, who suggested that a diet rich in soy foods may be the primary reason why "hot flashes and other menopausal symptoms are so infrequent in Japanese women." Japanese women also have lower rates of heart disease and breast cancer than Western women, which many researchers attribute to their soy-rich diets. Several researchers in the United States are currently investigating whether soy foods can ease menopausal symptoms in western women.

Q. *Several years ago I took birth control pills and immediately developed a nasty and vaginal yeast infection, so I discontinued using them. It took several months for me to get rid of the infection. Now that I am postmenopausal, my doctor suggested that I take estrogen replacement therapy. I am worried, however, that estrogen will worsen my yeast problem. Will taking estrogen once again trigger a yeast infection?*

A. A healthy vagina is a slightly acidic environment in which many different types of microscopic organisms thrive. So-called good bacteria in the vagina help to prevent the overgrowth of candida albicans, the fungus responsible for yeast infections. In the past, birth control pills contained very high doses of estrogen, which did appear to alter the normal acidic environment in the vagina, thus promoting yeast infections. The doses of estrogen that are used today in birth control pills and in hormone replacement therapy are much lower and do not appear to alter the normal acidic balance in the vagina. Preliminary studies indicate that these low doses of estrogen should not increase the risk of contracting a yeast infection.

Q. *Since I've been taking HRT (estrogen and progesterone) I've noticed that I've lost all interest in sex. Could the hormones be causing a loss in sex drive?*

A. Most women experience just the opposite reaction on HRT; they find that it actually enhances their sex drive. In your case, however, you may be having an adverse reaction to the progesterone component of your therapy, which could dampen libido in some women. I recommend that you talk to your gynecologist about reducing your progesterone dose, or taking a different type of pill altogether. According to the latest studies, simply adding a small amount of the male hormone to the female hormones normally used in HRT could enhance libido, and in fact, some doctors are already prescribing this combination pill to their patients. A word of caution: In some women, the HDL drops to dangerous levels with even small amounts of testosterone; I've had to discontinue it for this reason in some of my patients.

Q. *I have had breast cancer and am now going through menopause. I'm having such bad hot flashes at night that I'm losing sleep and I'm exhausted. I know I cannot take HRT, and the so-called natural remedies have not worked. Do I have any other options?*

A. Two drugs, clonidine and megestrol acetate (Megace), have been shown to help to control hot flashes and can be used by women with a history of breast cancer. Talk to your doctor to see if either of these would be helpful to you.

Q. *I am a divorced woman who has been abstinent for several years. I am now several dating someone and will be beginning a sexual relationship. I'm not on HRT. Is there anything I need to know about sex after menopause?*

A. After a long period of abstinence, it's only natural to be a bit anxious about resuming a sexual relationship. Sex can be every bit as rewarding after menopause as before, and in fact, many women find sex after menopause to be even better because they are no longer worried about becoming pregnant. There have been some changes in your body, however, of which you should be aware. In particular, when estrogen levels dip after menopause, the vaginal lining can become thin and dry, and the vagina can lose some of its flexibility and tone, which can make intercourse uncomfortable. Regular sexual activity (either through intercourse or masturbation) will help maintain the vaginal lining and flexibility. Estrogen replacement therapy can prevent these changes from occurring in the first place.

Since you are not taking estrogen, you will need to take other steps to prepare for sexual activity. I recommend that you use a topical estrogen cream (your doctor will have to prescribe this for you) in your vagina for at least two weeks prior to intercourse to build up the lining and restore tone. If this is not an option for you, you can use an over-the-counter vaginal moisturizer instead. You will find many different types of these at your local drugstore. Usually, these creams are sold in premeasured packages that are inserted into the vagina just as you would a tampon. The usual dose is one premeasured package every other day.

Second, since you have not been sexually active for several years, your vaginal cavity may be tight and contracted. You can start preparing for intercourse by dilating your vagina: Simply insert a well-lubricated finger, then two, into the vaginal cavity. You can also use a smooth-tipped vibrator to dilate the vagina. If the vaginal cavity feels very tight, you should consult with your gynecologist to see if further treatment is needed. If the vaginal area has atrophied to the point that normal remedies will not work, your doctor may prescribe hormone replacement therapy, at least until the vaginal lining has been built up. In addition, when you are actually having intercourse, keep in mind that lubrication may take longer, and you may need to use an artificial lubricant such as K-Y Jelly (saliva also works well) if necessary to help penetration.

Menopausal women often find that orgasm is not as intense as before. Nevertheless, multiple or sustained orgasm is possible to achieve if that was the case for you before menopause.

Although you may no longer be capable of becoming pregnant, you still need to be concerned about contracting a sexually transmitted disease. Unless you are involved in a long-term, monogamous relationship with someone you know very well and trust, you must insist that your partner use a latex condom. Most reasonable people will consent to HIV testing before starting a long-term relationship, and it is entirely appropriate to ask a prospective mate to have this done—particularly when you yourself are willing to be tested, too.

Q. *Do men go through a type of menopause? Lately, my husband's mood swings (he has just turned fifty) seem worse than mine!*

A. Oddly enough, I am asked this question more often by women than by men. I suspect this is because women may notice subtle changes in the men in their lives as they age, and unlike the female menopause, there is no handy label to affix to these changes.

As they get older, men do experience both physical and emotional changes. Some of these changes may not be quite as dramatic as they are in women, but they are definitely real. For example, by the time a man reaches his fifth decade, there is a small but steady decline in the production of testosterone, the male sex hormone. Although a man may remain fertile throughout his entire life, erections and orgasm often become harder to achieve, and many middle-aged and older men find that they need visual and auditory stimuli more than they did when they were younger. Women often misinterpret this as a sign that their partners are no longer interested in them. Many women have told me, "My husband won't have sex anymore unless he reads

Penthouse or watches a dirty movie before coming to bed," and their tone often suggests that they are hurt that their husbands no longer find them stimulating. I think that better understanding of the sexual changes men are experiencing could help reduce these hurt feelings and improve communication between partners.

For men, middle age may also usher in a period of reevaluation of their lives. As their bodies age, many men become aware of their mortality, particularly if their fathers died young. I have had men in my office literally panicked by the anniversary of a father's death—they are both apprehensive about approaching the same age and guilty when they live through the birthday themselves. These emotions are not unlike those that women experience during menopause. Women are encouraged to talk about these feelings (just look at all the books that have been written on menopause), but there is a deafening silence when it comes to the so-called male menopause. I'd suggest that a husband with the "dwindles" see his internist for a measurement of both his testosterone and yes—his estrogen—levels. The most knowledgeable male physicians I know are monitoring their own hormonal levels and some are actually taking replacement testosterone to keep their muscle mass and sense of vitality in top form. As we continue to learn about the multiple sites of action of estrogen in the body (the brain, the liver, the skin, etc.), particularly in stabilizing the contractile activity of the vasculature, researchers are beginning to consider how estrogen might be given to men whose levels are dangerously low. Men's estrogen levels are usually about 50 picamoles/dl.; this is a higher level than that of a postmenopausal woman, who not infrequently has levels of 30 or lower!

Menstrual Problems

Q. *My periods are so painful that I often need to spend a day or two in bed. My doctor said that it was normal for some women to experience a lot of discomfort, but I'm wondering if he's right. Is it normal?*

A. The medical term for menstrual pain is dysmenorrhea, and it is a very common complaint. Although some menstrual discomfort is normal, it is definitely abnormal for a woman to be in such pain during her menstrual period that she needs to take to her bed. I recommend that you seek a second opinion from another gynecologist who is knowledgeable about the causes of and treatment for dysmenorrhea. To find the right doctor, you can either call the department of obstetrics and gynecology at a local medical school or teaching hospital, or ask a friend for a referral. When you finally meet with the doctor, be prepared to provide a precise description of when the pain occurs during your cycle, what it feels like, and what, if anything, relieves it. (For example, does it feel better when you're lying down, sitting, or standing? Does lying on your stomach help or hurt? Does aspirin help?) Your observations along with a thorough physical examination by the doctor will help provide valuable clues about what could be causing the pain. Depending on your diagnosis, your physician will devise an appropriate treatment program. In most cases, menstrual cramps can be relieved by taking a nonsteroidal anti-inflammatory drug like Advil or Aleve. These over-the-counter medications will stop the production of prostaglandins, hormones that trigger uterine contractions and cause the severe cramps. A caveat: Excessive menstrual bleeding may follow taking one of these preparations. Some women may find relief by taking a diuretic, or "water pill," to rid the body of excess salt and water, which contribute to the often described feeling of bloating and abdominal distention. Regular exercise has also been shown to reduce menstrual cramps (although I would avoid doing abdominal crunches on the days you are most prone to menstrual pain). For many women, avoiding salt and caffeine before their menstrual periods may also be helpful. If your doctor suspects that a hormonal imbalance may be responsible for the pain, she may prescribe oral contraceptives to correct the imbalance or to block ovulation.

There are more serious reasons for menstrual pain, and these should certainly be investigated by your doctor. About 2 percent of all women have endometriosis, a condition in which cells normally confined to the uterine lining are implanted throughout the pelvic cavity and begin to grow in the ovaries, bladder, fallopian tubes, or between the rectum and the vagina. These misplaced cells bleed during the menstrual cycle, which can be quite painful. Endometriosis can be controlled through hormone therapy or corrected with laparoscopic surgery.

Severe menstrual cramps can also be a symptom of a pelvic inflammatory infection. It is possible to be harboring an infection without even knowing it, although some women may experience symptoms such as fever, chills, and a vaginal discharge. Infections can be treated successfully with antibiotics, and once the infection is under control, the pain usually disappears. Painful periods may also be due to fibroid tumors, benign growths in the uterus. Fibroids can be treated either surgically or medically, depending on their type and size.

Q. *I frequently spot in between my periods. Is this a sign of a problem? What could be causing it?*

A. By "spotting," I assume you mean that you are finding vestiges of blood on your underwear when you are not menstruating, which you believe is from your reproductive tract. However, don't jump to any conclusions: It's often difficult for a patient to precisely pinpoint where the blood is coming from. For example, I've had patients who were absolutely convinced that they were spotting menstrual blood when, it fact, the blood was due to bleeding hemorrhoids. That is why it is essential to be examined by a physician to determine the actual origin of the bleeding. Keep in mind that bleeding could also be a sign of pelvic inflammatory disease, an infection of the uterus or the fallopian tubes, a vaginal lesion, cervical polyps, or any number of other problems including cancer that are not necessarily related to the menstrual cycle.

The quantity and color of blood may be important clues about the source of the bleeding. A light stain of dark brown blood is a markedly different symptom than a gush of fresh, red blood. Be sure to tell your physician the type of bleeding that you are experiencing. In younger women, spotting between periods is often due to hormonal imbalance. Your gynecologist can check whether your estrogen/progesterone cycling is normal. If the levels of hormones are too low, she may recommend oral contraceptives to stabilize the cycle. Spotting can also be a sign of an early miscarriage. If you have been trying to get pregnant, and have noticed frequent mid-cycle spotting, you should bring it to the attention of your gynecologist. You may be low in certain hormones that are necessary to sustain a pregnancy, and may require hormone therapy.

After menopause, spotting is most often a sign of fibroid tumors, cancers of the endometrial lining of the uterus, or an excess of synthetic estrogen.

In sum, if you notice any blood coming from your vagina or rectal area, call your doctor for a complete examination.

Q. *About a week before my period, I feel bloated and irritable. Is this normal? Do I have PMS?*

A. Premenstrual syndrome (PMS) is one of the most common complaints of menstruating women, yet it is one of the most poorly understood of all medical problems. It is even difficult to find an authoritative definition of PMS: Different symptoms appear in different women and many even vary in the same woman from cycle to cycle. Similarly, the same woman may experience near incapacitating PMS before some periods, while others are virtually symptom-free. Therefore, PMS is broadly defined as a constellation of disturbing changes in body weight, sensation, and mood. Generally, PMS begins after ovulation, usually appearing within a week to ten clays before the menstrual blood begins to flow. The symptoms may intensify as the time of menstruation approaches and include one or more of the following:

- psychological changes including depression, irritability, anxiety, and/or changes in sleep habits and libido

- breast tenderness
- nausea, diarrhea, or abdominal bloating
- headache
- pelvic pain or cramping

The precise cause of PMS is unknown. Some of the possible culprits that have been considered include:

- fluctuation in the levels of hormones produced by the ovaries, which include estrogen, progesterone, and others
- a change in brain chemicals (neurotransmitters) as a result of monthly hormonal changes
- a change in the salt and water balance to ovarian steroids (hormones).

Depending on the symptoms of PMS, physicians can offer the following remedies:

- If you suffer from water retention, weight gain, and leg or ankle swelling, ask your physician for a mild diuretic ("water pill"); you can take a diuretic for one or two days before your period. (Only use a diuretic under a doctor's supervision; the excessive use of water pills can be very dangerous.)
- Some studies suggest that breast tenderness may be relieved by an herbal remedy, evening primrose oil, which is sold in both pharmacies and natural-food stores. For severe cases, your physician may prescribe bromocriptine (2.5 mg. at bedtime) or even danazol (200 gm. daily).
- For depression, difficulty concentrating, or other mental or emotional problems, your physician may prescribe vitamin B6 (pyridoxine) for short periods and in small doses (50-100 mg. daily). Although B6 may be helpful, it can cause serious nerve damage and should not be used unless under a physician's supervision.
- Pelvic pain may be relieved by any number of nonsteroidal anti-inflammatory drugs (Aleve, Advil, Motrin) that prevent the synthesis of prostaglandins, hormonelike substances that can cause uterine cramping. Simple, over-the-counter non-steroidal anti-inflammatory drugs (NSAIDs) are often effective. Do not exceed the recommended dosage; large doses of these drugs can result in excessive menstrual bleeding.
- As a last resort, if nothing helps, your physician may prescribe a drug known as gonadotrophic releasing hormone antagonist that blocks your ovarian cycles altogether. Given in combination with small doses of

estrogen, to prevent estrogen deficiency, this drug is now being tried in patients with extreme and severe symptoms.

If you suspect that you have PMS, keep a diary of your symptoms for three or four months. Be sure to carefully track when your symptoms appear, and which ones are the most bothersome. This information will help your physician tailor the therapy to counter your specific problems. Keep in mind that adequate sleep, good nutrition, and regular exercise have all been shown to relieve PMS and painful menstrual cramping.

A final word: Almost half of all patients have reported PMS improvement when taking a placebo (a pill with no known therapeutic action). This doesn't mean that the symptoms are all "in your head." The placebo, or feeling that you are doing something positive to help your symptoms, may actually cause a change in the brain's chemistry that may relieve some of what you are feeling. Simply because the symptom is not understood does not mean that it is not real. If your physician refuses to take your complaints seriously, find another doctor!

Mental Health

Q. *My husband and I split up a year ago. When we initially broke up, I was relieved and happy to finally be free of what had become a very tense relationship. Now that the divorce is finalized, however, I find I am so depressed that I'm having trouble functioning. I am normally a productive and happy person, but now, even the smallest task seems to be overwhelming, and sometimes I break out in tears for no reason at all. I have two small children and a full-time job, and, frankly, I do not have the time or the financial resources to slow down. I also would like to remarry one day, but I'm in no condition to go on a date. Should I ask my doctor to prescribe an antidepressant? Should I give myself a few more weeks to see if I feel better before seeking help?*

A. Although I cannot offer a definitive diagnosis, based on what you are telling me, you may very well be showing signs of depression. Given your situation, I think your reaction is perfectly normal. Once the reality of a divorce sets in, it is only natural to mourn the end of what was once a loving relationship, and to be uncertain about what the future may hold. In your case, you are also overwhelmed by the prospect of having to raise children, work full-time, and renegotiate a social life—and your children may be downright hostile about the demands of this last item and its implications for them.

I urge you to see your doctor, but not for the sole purpose of getting a pill that will magically make your problems disappear. Putting your marriage behind you and making a new life for yourself is going to take time, and no drug can accelerate this healing process. You will need to work it through, but this does not mean you need to work it through alone. If you were my patient, I would first do a thorough examination to make sure there were no physical problems causing your depression. (Even though I may believe that your depression is linked to your divorce, a good doctor does not take anything for granted.) For example, an underactive thyroid gland, which is a common condition in women, could drain you of your energy and make you feel anxious and sad. So can a significant anemia. Barring any obvious physical problem, I would then try to spend some time listening to your concerns and helping you work through verbalizing some of what most frightens you and what you find most upsetting. This can vary tremendously from woman to woman. Some rejoice at being alone but fear financial ruin. Others long for a new partner and worry about how long it will be before they find a sexual and emotional partner again. If this doesn't provide some relief and my patient makes no progress, I'd refer you to a carefully selected psychiatrist for psychiatric counseling. A psychiatrist (or psychologist) can best determine the kind of treatment that you may require. In many cases, simply talking about your feelings in a therapeutic environment may be most helpful and will provide you with the insight you need to better cope with your problems. In fact, some studies show that the "talking cure" is every bit as effective as medication. If your psychiatrist determines you need an antidepressant, however, she will prescribe one.

There are several different types of depressive disorders. The kind of depression you may be experiencing is called a "reactive depression"—that is, it is in response to a personal tragedy or event that evokes powerful emotions of anxiety and sadness, in your case, your divorce. What is bewildering about a reactive depression is that it may strike someone who has never been depressed before, which can make these feelings all the more threatening. At times, depression may afflict a patient for no apparent reason; there is no event of life change that precipitates the depression—it seems to strike out of the blue. This is called an endogenous depression and the symptoms often persist for weeks or even months before the patient finally seeks help.

When to get help Depression is a very treatable problem, but it is often difficult to get people in for treatment. Many people simply do not know when it is appropriate to ask for professional help. According to the American Psychiatric Association, if you have four or more of the following symptoms continuously for more than two weeks, you should seek medical help:

- change in appetite or weight
- change in sleep pattern
- loss of energy and feeling tired
- loss of pleasure in things that you used to enjoy
- overwhelming feelings of sadness or grief, especially if you are worse in the morning or are waking up hours earlier than usual
- feelings of hopelessness
- feelings of guilt
- inability to concentrate or think clearly
- recurrent thoughts of death or suicide
- disturbed thinking not rooted in reality; feeling, for example, that you are being punished because you have committed a terrible sin.

I do not believe that you necessarily have to have four of these symptoms to seek help. If your life is being disrupted by your depression to the point that it is interfering with your quality of life, I recommend that you get treatment.

Q. *What is the difference between depression and anxiety? (I think I may be suffering from both.)*

A. Although they may occur simultaneously, depression and anxiety are considered two different psychiatric disorders. Recently, psychiatrists have grouped emotional disorders characterized by heightened anxiety into the umbrella category of anxiety disorders. These are all characterized by heightened tension and include not only panic disorder, but five other distinct syndromes:

Generalized anxiety disorder This disorder is characterized by unrealistic worries about yourself, others, or your life situation. Patients may have a generalized fear that something is wrong, or that a loved one will come to some harm. Even when specific worries are not present, the patient is troubled by a constant sense of heightened tension or edginess.

Phobias A phobia is an intense fear of social situations, objects, or of being either alone or in a public place where you cannot escape. For example, in the case of agoraphobia, people may be terrified at the thought of leaving their home. I had one patient tell me it took all of her courage just to leave her apartment and get into the elevator each morning.

Panic attacks The person who suffers from panic attacks experiences overwhelming feelings of terror that do not have any apparent cause. The sufferer may sweat profusely, feels her heart beating wildly, and gasps for air. Often, the patient believes she is dying, or at the very least losing her mind. Many individuals who suffer panic attacks have higher levels of stress hormones that keep them in a state of alertness, particularly norepinephrine. (Panic attacks are more common in patients who suffer from an otherwise seldom serious disorder of the heart, mitral valve prolapse, than the rest of the population. For more information, see the Heart section, beginning on page 126.)

Obsessive compulsive disorder This condition is characterized by recurrent and unpleasant thoughts or a compulsion to repeat a series of acts (washing your hands, repeating words or a group of words over and over, or counting objects you see as you walk along a street, etc.).

Post-traumatic stress disorder This can occur after a shocking or traumatic event. Characteristic symptoms include general anxiety, guilt, difficulty thinking or concentrating, an excessive tendency to be startled by ordinary stimuli, inability to enjoy people or activities that were once pleasurable, nightmares, or vivid memories of the events that caused trouble. (Sometimes the memory is so vivid that the sufferer believes he is reliving the event.)

In reality, there is often an overlap between depression and anxiety, and many patients show symptoms of both. Some patients may have what is called an "agitated depression," which is defined as an unpleasant tension that may at times burgeon into attacks of unmanageable panic. These symptoms are so troublesome that they may prevent the patient from thinking clearly, and many may not be able to perform their jobs.

Both depression and anxiety appear to run in families, and although both problems may be caused by variations in the processing of certain chemicals by the brain, many psychiatrists believe that these are in part learned behaviors. In other words, if you are raised by someone who is continually depressed or easily thrown into a panic, you may actually learn this behavior.

There are very effective medications for both depression and anxiety disorders; often, more than one medication is necessary for these combined ailments.

Q. *I am very shy. Can Prozac give me a better personality?*

A. There is no question that fluoxetine (Prozac) is a remarkable drug for many people and that it is very effective in alleviating depressive mood and reducing anxiety with minimum side effects. Prozac is part of a class of drugs known as serotonin reuptake inhibitors. It works on serotonin, a hormone in the brain that does not appear to be produced normally in many depressed people. As with any psychotropic medication, however, Prozac must be prescribed judiciously. In recent years, there have been many books and magazine articles touting the benefits of Prozac, and this has led to a great deal of misunderstanding about what this drug can and cannot do. Many of these books and articles describe how Prozac has quite literally transformed the personalities of those who are taking it; in fact, in one best-selling book, *Listening to Prozac*, the author, who is a psychiatrist, describes case study after case study of patients whose lives were vastly improved by simply popping this one little pill. Typically, patients went from being shy, angry, withdrawn, and unfulfilled individuals to warm, happy, loving, and outgoing people. I am not sure, though, that this is really a happy ending. In my opinion, redesigning personalities is not the role of the medical profession. It is one thing to change pathologic or psychotic behavior that causes unbearable suffering for either the patient or society; it is quite another to use medication to achieve a "better personality." The purpose of Prozac (or any antidepressant) is simply to help you take better charge of the situations in your life that are making you unhappy. At times, if a patient is so depressed and anxious that she unable to function, Prozac is a useful tool (to be prescribed on a temporary basis) to better help her concentrate on working through her problems. Prozac is not a cure; the problems in your life will persist unless you learn to deal with them in a more constructive way.

I had the opportunity to listen to a very thoughtful psychiatrist, an expert in prescribing psychotropic medications, discussing his ethical concerns about using these drugs. He believed that Prozac was in a different category than any of the other antidepressant medications, and believed that it actually did produce a real change in the essential personality or *anima* (the spiritual nature or essential force of a person) of the individual on the medication. He felt that deliberately setting out to do this with drugs was a serious ethical problem that has not been adequately addressed.

Apart from ethical considerations, there are some serious problems with Prozac. The "quick fix" promised by this and similar medications negates, in a way, the value of suffering and conflict in making people develop adaptive mechanisms and coping skills they would not otherwise have. In other words, you learn nothing by taking the drug unless it is combined with a good therapeutic program. One of the most important uses of antidepressants is to enable the patient to participate in psychotherapy—to find ways of expressing the nature of his or her suffering and to design with an expert counselor ways of coping with psychic illness and pain. Prozac and the other newer antidepressants are incompletely tested in the long term, and we do not know their long-term effects. We do know that after some people are on Prozac for two to four years, for example, they seem to develop less sensitivity to the medication and may require either a "drug holiday" or a higher dose to get the same result. The higher the dose, the more likelihood of unpleasant side effects such as sleepiness and excessive fatigue. Another unwelcome consequence of Prozac, by the way, is that it makes orgasm difficult or even impossible to achieve for both men and women.

My advice is that before you agree to pop a pill find out whether it is possible to achieve the same result through psychotherapy. Although it may take longer, the effect may be longer lasting, and it is not dependent on taking medication. If you do take Prozac, I would not advise using it on a long-term basis unless everything else has failed.

Q. *I cannot make it to work in the morning without turning back at least once or twice on my way to the car to check that the oven is off or that I unplugged the coffeemaker. Is this a sign of compulsive behavior?*

A. Given the fact that many of us are very rushed in the morning, it is not unreasonable for someone to feel compelled to double-check that the appliances are turned off, the faucets are not dripping, or that the cat is not locked out of the house. If after double-checking (or even triple-checking) you are then able to leave for work and function well throughout the day, I would not call your behavior abnormal. There are people, though, who simply cannot stop checking. Typically, they take a few steps out of the door, and then feel compelled to turn back and recheck everything all over again, often repeating their actions scores of times. As a result, they are late for appointments and are unable to perform such basic tasks as holding a job or picking their children up from school. This type of behavior is typical of an obsessive-compulsive disorder that is characterized by the repetition of a complex ritual for no apparent reason. Other examples of obsessive-compulsive disorders may be the continual washing of hands, often until they bleed, or an inability to get rid of a weird or bizarre thought. Although people with obsessive-compulsive behavior often recognize the irrationality of their behavior or thoughts, they appear to have no control over themselves. As bizarre as obsessive-compulsive disorders may appear, they are actually quite common and can be easily treated with small doses of antidepressant medication.

Q. *Since my husband died, I have seen or spoken to him several times, often at night. I'm certain that his visits are real, yet I know they cannot be. Am I losing my mind?*

A. I have a dear friend who confided in me that she often visited with her dead father, whom she "truly" saw and to whom she "truly" spoke, particularly when she was troubled or stressed. She knew that these "apparitions" were not real, but she derived great comfort from them anyway. Such "appearances" (which a sane person understands at least intellectually cannot be genuine) are mechanisms by which our minds defend against the overwhelming grief

171

of an irrevocable loss. The clue here is when you say, "I'm certain that his visits are real, yet I know they cannot be." As much as you may want to believe that your husband is back with you, you know he is not.

Many patients come to me with similar concerns; typically, they have been communicating with a dead child, spouse, parent, or friend and they need to know if they are showing signs of mental illness. I simply listen calmly and try to decide whether the patient understands that such appearances cannot be real. If we agree that the "visitations" are not disturbing but comforting, and that they do not become so dominant or intrusive that the patient or others are disturbed by them, I reassure the patient that what she is experiencing is perfectly normal under the circumstances.

Q. I have been under a lot of stress lately. My mother passed away recently, my husband has started a new business, and I am under a great deal of pressure at work. I told my doctor that I was feeling "stressed out" and he wrote out a prescription for Valium. My older brother and I use the same doctor. I was talking to my brother and found out that he, too, went to the doctor complaining of stress-related symptoms, but in his case, the doctor recommended that he join a gym and sent him to a special program on stress control run at our local hospital. I can't help feeling that I was being dismissed as a "hysterical female" while my brother's complaints were taken more seriously because he's male. Could I be right?

A. Without knowing the medical history of both you and your brother it is difficult for me to make a snap judgment. I do know, however, that 70 percent of all prescriptions for psychotropic medication written in the United States are for women, and although there may be times when the use of tranquilizers are legitimate, I have personally seen many cases in which tranquilizers were prescribed for women who either did not really need them or had other physical problems that went undetected. For example, in one case, a rapid heartbeat in a young woman was misdiagnosed as a sign of anxiety when in reality it was due to the existence of an extra muscle pathway between the upper and lower chambers of her heart. Several studies have documented that physicians—especially male physicians—are more likely to see women as more emotional or hysterical than men, and women too often believe that their symptoms are "all in their head" or the result of emotional problems. The combination of prejudice in the mind of the physician and the patient herself about women's greater emotional vulnerability helps promote this unfortunate situation.

This is not to say that tranquilizers are bad drugs—not at all. Valium and related compounds are invaluable aids for patients with abnormal or pernicious anxiety over the short term. If anxiety is persistent or incapacitating, the patient needs the attention of a competent psychiatrist who will assess the mental or emotional disorder responsible for the anxiety and/or depression and prescribe the drug that would be most useful for the patient. I think the habit of the general practitioner to prescribe the "latest" antianxiety medication without consultation or special education by a competent psychopharmacologist is downright dangerous.

It can also be dangerous if a physical ailment is neglected because the physician is convinced that the symptoms are emotional. There are ways that a patient can tell whether her physician has carefully considered her case, whether the diagnosis of an emotional problem may be appropriate, and whether a psychotropic drug should be considered. I do not believe that any prescription for any medication—psychotropic or not—should be written until the doctor has fully examined the patient. There is no way that a doctor can determine if a problem is emotional if she has not ruled out the physical possibilities. If a doctor begins to write a prescription for a tranquilizer, it is within a patient's right to ask, "What makes you believe that I do not have a real organic disease? On what data are you basing this decision?" Although some doctors may be a bit defensive about being questioned, I think the majority will be relieved to have this kind of discussion; often it can clear the air. If you are still convinced that the doctor has not properly diagnosed your problem, you should ask for copies of your records so that you can get a second opinion.

If you and your doctor determine that your symptoms are emotional or psychiatric in origin, it is advisable to seek counseling from a psychologist or psychiatrist before taking any medication. There are often better ways to control stress than by simply taking a pill. In fact, many hospitals and health centers have special stress clinics that specialize in teaching people the techniques and skills necessary to cope with stress.

Nails

Q. *My nails are very soft and are constantly chipping and breaking. This is not only unattractive, but it can be painful I get regular manicures, but they do not seem to help. I'm considering using artificial nails but I'm worried that they'll make my nails worse. Could they? Is there anything I can do to make my nails stronger?*

A. The condition you are describing—soft, peeling, splitting nails—is called brittle nail syndrome and it is one of the most common of all nail problems. I asked my associate Dr. Richard Scher, who is a dermatologist and a specialist in nail disorders, how to treat this problem. Here are his recommendations.

Basic nail care In order to understand how to care for your nails, you need to understand a bit about how they grow. The growth of the nail plate (the hard part of the nail) is controlled by the nail's matrix, or growth center, which extends from the moon shaped lower part of the nail to about one-quarter inch below the skin line. Any damage to the lower nail can result in damage to the growth center. Therefore, it is essential that the area around the growth center be handled very gently. It is not a good idea to cut the cuticle or push it down with a hard stick or sharp object, as is done by many professional manicurists. Instead, clean, polish-free nails should be soaked in warm water for about ten minutes. Apply a good moisturizer (any brand is fine). When the cuticle is soft, take a moist towel and gently push the excess skin away from the nail. Once the cuticle is pushed off the nail, it will dry up and fall off.

When washing your nails, use a soft brush and avoid vigorous brushing, which can damage the growth center.

Nail polish can actually protect the nail bed and helps slow the loss of moisture. To prevent damage to nails, use only formaldehyde-free polish and acetone-free remover. Remove polish weekly. It is a good idea to let the nails go polish-free for one day each week so that they can breathe.

Be sure to wear gloves when washing dishes or doing housework to protect nails from potentially irritating cleaning agents.

Do not use your nails as tools (to screw in a nail or as a can opener) since a sharp blow to the nail can damage the growth center.

Vitamins Studies have shown that supplements of biotin, a B vitamin, can promote nail growth in many people. In one Swiss study, 300 mcg. of biotin were given to people with brittle nail syndrome three times daily. About 65 percent of all patients showed some improvement. Since 300 mcg. is a very high dose of biotin, and even though there have been no reported cases of any untoward effects, Dr. Scher advises taking this vitamin under the supervision of your physician.

Acrylic nails According to Dr. Scher, acrylic nails are okay as long as you are not allergic to the acrylic and follow some basic guidelines. First, these nails must be removed every three months for at least a week to give the nails time to breathe. If left on indefinitely, moisture can gather under the nail bed, which can damage the real nail and be the perfect breeding ground for a fungal infection.

Fungal infections Any discolorization or yellowing of the nail could be a sign of a bacterial or fungal infection. Until recently, there have been few effective treatments for fungal infections of the nail, which can be quite persistent. Although there are several antifungal over-the-counter and prescription medications for topical use, they can take months or even years to completely cure the infection. The FDA has recently approved an antifungal agent (itraconazole), which can be taken orally, that has been shown to eliminate an infection of the toenails in four months, and an infection of the fingernails in two to three months. Two other antifungal medications (fluconazole and terbinafine) are expected to be approved by the FDA for this purpose within the year. If you have a fungal infection of the nail, talk to your doctor about these new treatments.

175

Osteoporosis

Q. *My mother has severe osteoporosis. As she got older, she lost several inches of height and by the time she was seventy, she looked like a bent, frail old lady. Last year, she broke her hip and is now in a nursing home. I am fifty, and have just become menopausal. My doctor tells me that I am also at high risk of developing osteoporosis. I do not want to end up like my mother. Is there anything I can do to prevent this from happening to me? (I do take calcium pills every day, but my grandmother had breast cancer so I am reluctant to take hormone replacement therapy.)*

A. First, the good news. There have recently been some exciting new break-throughs in the treatment of osteoporosis that, for the first time, may allow doctors to treat this "bone breaking" disease effectively. The bad news is, osteoporosis appears to be hereditary, and if your mother or grandmother had it, you have a good chance of getting it, too.

About half of all women over the age of fifty will develop osteoporosis—the thinning and wearing away of bone—which increases their susceptibility to breaks and fractures. Small-boned, slender Caucasian and Asian women are at greatest risk of developing osteoporosis. Women who are heavy drinkers (more than two alcoholic beverages daily) and smoke are also at a higher risk of becoming osteoporotic.

The gradual loss of bone is a normal part of the aging process and it happens to both men and women. Osteoporosis, however, is due to an accelerated loss of bone and it affects three times as many women as men. This rapid loss of bone, which begins after menopause, is believed to be caused by the decline in estrogen, a hormone that is essential for the absorption of calcium, a key mineral in bone formation. During childhood and early adulthood, old bone is continually being replaced by new bone until we develop our peak bone mass at around age thirty. At that point, the production of new bone begins to slow down, and old bone begins to wear away. After menopause, the rate of bone loss begins to speed up. In fact, women begin to lose 2-4 percent of their bone mass annually for about a decade, when the loss begins to level off. Some women lose bone at an even faster rate, making them especially vulnerable to fractures.

Studies have shown that most women underestimate the seriousness of this problem; in fact, three out of four postmenopausal women have never discussed osteoporosis with their doctors. Women clearly do not view bone loss with the same urgency as they do cancer or even heart disease. This can be a serious mistake. About 40 percent of all postmenopausal women will develop vertebral fractures that can result in the rounded back or "dowager's hump." More than 300,000 women will get hip fractures, which not only leave many women permanently disabled but can be deadly: about 20 percent of all women who fracture their hips die within six months of the injury due to complications such as pneumonia.

Fortunately, there are many things that can be done to reduce your risk of developing osteoporosis, or to prevent a mild case from turning into a serious one.

Getting an accurate diagnosis Given the prevalence of osteoporosis, it is advisable for every woman to have a bone density test at around the time of menopause. The fastest and most accurate test is the dual-energy X-ray absorptiometry (DXA or DEXA). During this test, the patient lies on a table and an X-ray machine takes a picture of her skeleton. From this simple and painless procedure, the doctor can determine early signs of excessive bone loss and can prescribe the appropriate treatment.

Calcium and Vitamin D Calcium is essential for strong bones, yet most women get only a fraction of the calcium they need through diet. Dietary calcium is more easily absorbed than supplements, so it's important to eat as many calcium-rich foods as possible. Low-fat dairy products, leafy green vegetables, and canned salmon or sardines with bones are calcium-rich foods. Although it is not a cure for osteoporosis, there is some evidence that calcium supplements combined with vitamin D can help slow bone loss. Women who are not on hormone replacement therapy should take 1,500 mg. of calcium daily with 400 IU of vitamin D; those who are on HRT should take 1,000 mg. of calcium daily with 400 IU of vitamin D. There are many different forms of calcium on the market; calcium citrate is one of the best absorbed.

Exercise Weight-bearing exercise (walking, jogging, running) can help maintain bone mass. A little exercise goes a long way: According to a recent study, women who walk as little as one mile a day show significantly less bone loss than nonwalkers, especially in their legs and torso. Interestingly, although Japanese women consume little calcium and are also at high risk of osteoporosis, the incidence of hip fractures in Japan is half that of the United States. The reason? Researchers suspect it's because Japanese women often sit on the floor, and the action of getting up and down throughout the day may exercise their hip bones.

Hormone replacement therapy Estrogen replacement therapy is one of the few treatments approved by the FDA for osteoporosis. Although estrogen does not promote bone growth, it does appear to slow the loss of bone and has been shown to prevent osteoporosis in many women. In fact, according to recent studies, estrogen can reduce the risk of fractures by about 50 percent. More important, estrogen can help prevent fractures even in cases of already established osteoporosis.

As I have noted earlier in this book, HRT is not appropriate for everybody. If a woman is considered to be at high risk of breast cancer—that is, if her mother, sibling, or grandmother had the disease—her doctor may not want to put her on HRT. Some doctors believe that osteoporosis can be so devastating, however, that for some women, HRT may be well worth the small increased risk of breast cancer.

Other Drugs If you cannot or do not want to take HRT, there are two new promising drugs that may be even more effective against osteoporosis.

Alendronate sodium (Fosamax) This drug was the first nonhormonal treatment approved by the FDA for osteoporosis. Available by prescription only, alendronate is one of a new class of drugs called the bisphosphonates. They work by slowing down the activity of cells called osteoclasts which resorb bone, thus allowing the activity of bone-building cells (osteoblasts) to dominate in the constant process of bone turnover. Like another medication that increases bone density, nasal calcitonin, alendronate seems to increase bone density for only a few years, and then apparently the situation stabilizes.

Fluoride and calcium A new, slow-release form of fluoride combined with calcium citrate has been shown to reduce spinal fractures and, more important, build bone in older women with severe osteoporosis. This is the first treatment for osteoporosis that has been proven to not only slow the loss of bone but to actually create new bone. Studies performed at the University of Texas Southwestern Medical Center followed women who were taking the fluoride calcium combination for three to four years. At the end of the treatment, bone mass in the women's spines grew by an average of 4-5 percent annually, and the density of the hip bones grew by more than 2 percent annually. The women in this study had far fewer spinal fractures than women with osteoporosis who were only taking calcium, and suffered significantly less back pain. As of this writing, this drug is pending FDA approval and will be available by prescription only.

Polycystic Ovaries

Q. *My eighteen-year-old daughter was recently diagnosed with polycystic ovaries, and her doctor wants to give her hormones to correct the problem. Are these hormones dangerous? Is my daughter at risk for cancer? Will she ever be able to have children?*

A. During a normal menstrual cycle, a follicle or egg develops in the ovary and is released around mid-cycle—the period of ovulation—so that it can be fertilized. The entire process is controlled by a delicate interplay among several hormones. In the case of polycystic ovaries, a hormonal imbalance causes the ovaries to produce numerous follicles, but they are not fully developed. Instead of being released, the eggs remain in a kind of arrested growth state within the ovaries. Polycystic ovaries are characterized by irregular and infrequent menstrual periods, sometimes as few as three or four a year, and higher than normal levels of male hormones. When women with polycystic ovaries do have periods, they are often very heavy. Due to hormonal irregularities, some women with polycystic ovaries have increased body and facial hair, acne and weight gain. This condition is very common—at least 5-10 percent of all American girls and women have two or more traits that are common to this syndrome. Polycystic ovaries can be diagnosed with a sonogram or ultrasound examination of the ovaries.

Women with polycystic ovaries have an increased risk of cancer of the lining of the uterus or the endometrium. The reason is simple: Although they are producing eggs, which ready the lining for implantation after fertilization, they are not shedding the lining on a regular basis, as they would during a monthly menstrual cycle. The longer the lining is allowed to build up, the greater the risk of cancer. Therefore, it may be advisable to give these women a synthetic version of the hormone progesterone, which would trigger menstrual bleeding. Used judiciously, this hormone is not dangerous, and in fact, under these conditions, may be a true lifesaver in that it can prevent cancer.

Women with polycystic ovaries may experience some fertility problems, but they are not insurmountable: In fact, very often the condition is first diagnosed after a woman has tried unsuccessfully to get pregnant. Your daughter is fortunate enough to know about her condition, so that she and her doctor can plan ahead. Typically, if a woman has polycystic ovaries and is having trouble conceiving, her doctor may prescribe a fertility drug to stimulate ovulation.

The real threat to women with polycystic ovaries may not be cancer but heart disease. According to one groundbreaking study done at the University of Pittsburgh, young women with this problem appear to have "a male coronary heart disease risk profile," which means they do not enjoy the same protection against heart disease as do most other premenopausal women. In a study of 206 girls and women with polycystic ovaries, the Pittsburgh researchers found that many of these girls and women had many risk factors for heart disease not normally seen in younger women, including high insulin levels, high blood levels of LDL ("bad cholesterol"), high levels of triglycerides, high blood pressure, and an increased waist/hip ratio (excess fat around the abdominal area). Also, women with polycystic ovary syndrome often have some degree of high blood pressure. The researchers strongly advised women with this problem to try to reduce their risk of heart disease by leading a heart-healthy lifestyle—that is, not smoking, eating a low-fat diet, getting enough exercise, and watching their weight. Any girl or woman with polycystic ovaries should be carefully monitored by her gynecologist and general practitioner.

Pregnancy

Q. *I have just found out that I'm pregnant. I read that during pregnancy you shouldn't take any medication because it can harm the baby. Is this true? What if I get sick?*

A. During pregnancy, a mother-to-be should not take any medication unless it is under the supervision of her physician. Although not all drugs will do so, some will cross the placenta and harm the fetus. For example, lithium, which is a very effective medication for manic depressive illness, is teratogenic (causes malformations in the developing fetus) and patients on this medication must discontinue it during pregnancy. In general, physicians who take care of pregnant women try to adhere to the following guidelines:

- Avoid using new drugs on their pregnant patients.
- The physician will monitor the medical literature for reports of fetal abnormalities in women taking established medications.
- If the mother-to-be gets sick, the physician will treat her in such a way that it does not pose a threat to the fetus wherever possible.

Some chronic illnesses must be treated during pregnancy, such as hypertension and asthma. In treating the pregnant woman with high blood pressure, it is usually safe to continue her medications with one exception: the class of drugs called angiotensin-converting enzyme inhibitors (ACE inhibitors) like Vasotec should not be used; another category of medication has to be substituted. The drugs we use to control asthma (theophylline, beta-two agonist bronchodilators, and even steroids for managing acute and severe episodes of asthma) are all safe during pregnancy. Some, like theophylline, might be metabolized a little differently in the pregnant patient, so drug levels might have to be carefully monitored.

During pregnancy, you should never self-medicate: Always check with your physician before popping a pill.

Q. *I am in my seventh month of pregnancy and I'm always out of breath, why is this happening?*

A. Your breathlessness is probably being caused by the way you are carrying your baby. By the seventh month of pregnancy, the uterus is high in the abdomen, right under the chest. Particularly in the case of a first pregnancy, the abdominal wall is firm and in some women does not distend easily. The diaphragm, the large chest muscle that causes the lungs to expand and contract, may not be able to work as efficiently because of the added weight from the abdomen. Therefore, the lung expansion may be impaired, thus creating the breathlessness.

In some cases, however, the feeling of breathlessness can be caused by anemia, a condition that occurs when the cells are not getting enough oxygen and may be caused by a deficiency in iron, folic acid, or vitamin B12. (For more information on anemia during pregnancy, see the next question, and read the section on anemia, page 36.)

Q. *I am in my second trimester and I constantly feel exhausted and run down. Is this normal?*

A. No, it is most definitely not normal. Although it is quite common for pregnant women to tire more easily than other women, constant exhaustion and fatigue is a sign that something is amiss. In all likelihood, you are suffering from an anemia caused by a nutritional deficiency. The old adage that "the baby takes what it needs" even at the cost of the mother's nutrition and well-being is partially true (although if you neglect yourself enough, the baby won't thrive either). I know from personal experience what can happen if a mother-to-be is not getting enough nutrients. When I was pregnant, I decided that a "good diet" was enough to keep me healthy during my nine months. In spite of fresh fruits, salads, and plenty of red meat, I was so tired by my fifth month that I could barely stand up. In line in the doctors' cafeteria one day, I complained to a colleague, who bet me $10 that I was folate deficient—that is, deficient in the B vitamin folic acid. A blood test revealed that I was indeed, and a week of folic acid supplements restored my blood count to normal levels. From that point on, I began to pay strict attention to taking the proper supplements to augment the "good diet." I recommend that you see your doctor immediately (don't wait for your monthly visit) and tell her how you're feeling. She will take the appropriate tests and recommend the correct supplements.

Restless Leg Syndrome

Q. *For the past year, I have had great difficulty sleeping because, when I lay down in bed, my legs begin to throb and ache. I have no choice but to get out of bed and walk around, often for hours. I finally do fall asleep—when I'm exhausted-but I can only sleep for a few hours at a time before my legs start to bother me again. When I told my family doctor about my problem, he said that it was probably due to anxiety and prescribed a sleeping pill, which did not help. When I saw a neurologist for an unrelated problem with my eyes, however, and described my symptoms, he told me that I had restless leg syndrome and gave me the name of a specialist in this disorder.*

I have never heard of this problem and, evidently, neither has my doctor. What is it and what can I do about it?

A. Restless leg syndrome (RLS) is one of the most misunderstood and over-looked medical problems today. Although it affects 12 million people, many physicians are still unaware of this disorder and, like yours, often dismiss the telltale symptoms as a sign of too much stress or a case of run-of-the-mill insomnia. In reality, RLS is a bona fide neurological problem that has recently been designated as a movement disorder (Parkinson's disease, a degenerative neurological disorder, is also a movement disorder but is unrelated to RLS.) In women, symptoms often begin during pregnancy and may abate until menopause, after which they return with a vengeance. In fact, about 15 percent of the population over fifty has some form of RLS, and it is a virtual epidemic in nursing homes.

Symptoms of RLS are often described by patients as a "creepy, crawly feeling" or an "achy," "crampy," or "tingling" sensation in the calves. As the condition worsens, some patients may experience sharp pains similar to electric shocks in their legs every few seconds. Moving the legs and shifting positions can bring temporary relief, but once the movement stops, the symptoms return. Since RLS often strikes at night, its victims can become seriously sleep-deprived and depressed. To make matters worse, between 70 and 90 percent of all people with RLS have a related condition called PLMS (periodic limb movements in sleep), which are repetitive, jerky movements in the legs and sometimes arms that occur at intervals of fifteen to forty seconds. Between the two conditions, it is very difficult to get a good night's sleep. People who suffer from RLS during the day may find long car trips or even sitting at a desk for any extended time close to intolerable. I know of one woman whose RLS was so bad that her husband installed an exercise bicycle in the back of their family van so she could be cycling away during car trips!

What causes RLS? Symptoms are believed to be related to the way the body processes the chemical dopamine, which is produced by the brain (low levels of dopamine are also associated with Parkinson's disease). In severe cases of RLS, patients may be treated with L-dopa, a dopamine-containing drug that is also used to treat Parkinson's, or painkillers, antidepressants, and other drugs. Symptoms of RLS may also be triggered by circulatory problems, iron deficiency, or a deficiency in folic acid, a B vitamin, and also appears to run in families. In some cases, vitamin supplements have been reported to help to relieve symptoms.

Mild exercise also appears to help many RLS patients, although a too rigorous workout can actually bring on an attack. Some patients find relief by doing gentle leg stretches throughout the day. RLS was a relatively unknown condition until two women—RLS sufferers themselves—began a national support group called the Night Walkers in 1992. The group encourages research in RLS and has helped to raise public awareness about this problem. If you think you have RLS, you should call the neurology department or sleep research center at your local hospital or medical school for the name of a physician who is knowledgeable about the treatment and diagnosis of this problem. (For information on where to find a doctor in your area familiar with RLS, see Resources, page 225.)

Scared to Death

Q. *Family legend has it that my great-aunt dropped dead immediately after hearing that her husband had been in a fatal car accident. Can people die from sudden shock or after a particularly upsetting or frightening experience?*

A. What you're actually talking about is a phenomenon known as "sudden death syndrome." Extreme stress—especially fear—can disrupt normal heart rhythms, which can be lethal. In fact, several decades ago Walter Cannon, a famous Harvard medical physiologist, hypothesized that voodoo death wasn't caused by magic but by the victim's belief that the voodoo practitioner had real supernatural powers. Cannon reasoned that the "cursed" person's absolute conviction that he or she was about to die precipitated a tremendous surge of "flight or fight" hormones that caused a fatal disruption in the normal rhythm of the heart. Later studies have shown that this is indeed possible, and that anxiety can have a profoundly negative effect on the heart rhythm.

   Women are more at risk of sudden death syndrome than men due to physiological differences in the function of the heart. As a result of these differences, it is more likely that a sudden shock will destabilize the normal rhythm of a woman's heart, which could trigger a fatal arrhythmia. For this reason, women must be particularly vigilant about being screened for coronary artery disease so that if they do have a problem, it can be identified and treated before it becomes a lethal one. In particular, women should have an annual electrocardiogram (EKG), a noninvasive test that measures electrical activity in the heart. An EKG will detect abnormalities in the heartbeat. One condition that predisposes to sudden cardiac death is known as the "long Q-T syndrome," a descriptive term that has its origin in the fact that the interval between two sets of deflection in the electrocardiogram (which we call the QRS and the T wave of the complex) is abnormally prolonged. The problem runs in families and is being studied in depth by Milanese cardiologist Dr. Peter Schwartz, who has collected a list of families in whom the long Q-T syndrome occurs. This problem should be closely monitored by your physician; in some cases medication may be prescribed.

Secondhand Smoke

Q. *I'm a working mother with two children—a three-year-old daughter and a year-old son. Most of the time I'm feeling exhausted and stressed out. I'm a smoker, and although I know I should quit, given my frantic lifestyle I'm not sure I can. My mother, an ex-smoker herself, is constantly berating me about smoking in front of the children. I think she's being self-righteous and should leave me alone. Am I really hurting my children by smoking?*

A. Given the pressure that you're under, I can understand why you feel you can't quit smoking. I can also understand your annoyance with your mother, whose criticism, at least indirectly, questions your judgment as a parent. You need to understand, however, that every time you light up in your home, you are putting your children, your spouse, and even your pets at risk. Second hand smoke whether it is exhaled smoke or smoke from a burning cigarette, cigar, or pipe—contains more than four thousand substances, forty of which are known causes of cancer in humans or animals. In fact, the U.S. Environmental Protection Agency has classified secondhand smoke as a known carcinogen in humans and unequivocally states that it is responsible for several thousand cancer deaths a year in the United States. Other substances found in smoke are strong irritants that can cause asthma and respiratory infections. Infants and small children exposed to secondhand smoke are at increased risk of lower respiratory tract infections and ear infection. Studies show that these children have reduced lung function and are more prone to coughs, phlegm, and wheezing.

These are all compelling reasons why you should not be smoking in front of your children. If you must smoke, do so outside of your home and away from your family.

Sex

Q. *Is sex during menstruation risky?*

A. Many societies have taboos about sex during menstruation; for example, intercourse during menstruation is banned in the Old Testament and menstruating women deemed to be "unclean." In reality, menstrual blood is actually sterile and there is no way of knowing why or how this taboo came into being. Today, many women engage in sex during menstruation, and some actually find it more enjoyable than during other times for two reasons: First, there is an increase in pelvic circulation during this period of the menstrual cycle, and second, there is a drop in progesterone levels during menstruation, which increases libido in some women. Sex during menstruation is not dangerous for either the woman or her partner. Due to the fact that the cervix is slightly open during menstruation, there is a theoretical risk that a woman could be more prone to contracting an infection than at other times of her cycle, but few doctors believe this is true. The use of a condom, however, should significantly reduce the risk of infection.

It is a good idea to use a condom anyway. Do not assume that you cannot get pregnant while you are menstruating, especially if it is during the later days of your menstrual cycle. Whenever you have intercourse, there is always a risk of pregnancy and you need to use a reliable contraceptive. (I would not recommend that you use a diaphragm or a contraceptive sponge during menstruation; studies have shown that these may increase the risk of toxic shock syndrome.)

Q. *My husband and I sometimes engage in "rough play" during sex. Sometimes he ties me up and slaps me. This excites me, but I wonder whether this is normal. What is the difference between "rough play" and sexual abuse?*

A. When it comes to something as individual and idiosyncratic as sexual practices, it is hard to define "normal." Many people thrive on the excitement of conflict in their lives and require the same kind of stimulation in their sexual relationships. It is not uncommon for people to act out their personalities—their likes, their dislikes, and their neuroses—in the bedroom. Some people enjoy playing violent games in and out of the sexual arena. Some people prefer to be cast in a submissive role and others like to play a dominant role. Some people find that being beaten is sexually stimulating. Your question—where do you draw the line—is a good one. From a physician's point of view, there are clear-cut guidelines. First, no one should emerge from a sexual encounter with injuries. Tying someone up, even overpowering them, is acceptable if the confined person does not become fearful, feels trapped, or gets hurt. If overpowering requires blackening an eye or knocking out a tooth, it is no longer sexual play but physical abuse. There are emotional guidelines as well: No one should feel humiliated during or after the sexual encounter. There should be a clear understanding of just how far each partner will go to satisfy the other, and neither partner should be asked to do things that he or she finds degrading. If one partner is continually pushing the other into situations that are uncomfortable or even painful, it is a sign that this couple needs to seek outside counseling.

Q. *My husband and I used to have a terrific sex life, but lately, our sexual encounters are few and far between. We love each other, but between our jobs and our kids, we are always rushed and exhausted. By the time we have a moment alone, we are simply too tired for sex. What's wrong with us?*

A. Many of my patients—both male and female—have confessed with great sadness that they believe the sexual adventure that enlivened their marriage is over. Although they may be in loving relationships, they are concerned about their lack of sexual activity. Very often, one or both partners may feel that the other is no longer attracted to them, and this only adds to their anxiety.

192

When I hear this type of complaint from a patient, I usually ask the following three questions: Where do your children sleep at night? How often do you and your spouse go out by yourselves? Have you taken a vacation alone as a couple recently, and if so, what happened? Much too often I hear the following answers: (1) the children wander around all night, frequently ending up in bed with their parents; (2) the couple rarely goes out alone anymore; (3) if the couple was lucky enough to get away together, 90 percent of the time my patient will answer that the vacation was like a "second honeymoon," but once the vacation ended, she and her husband reverted back to their old habits.

What I have surmised from all of this is that, all too often, the pressures of daily living can encroach on even the best of marriages. People who work hard at their jobs and/or are raising children may have little left to give their partners at the end of the day. This does not mean that the marriage is not a solid one, or that the spouses are no longer interested in each other, but the fact that one or both partners may be upset by the lack of sex does indicate that there is a growing communication problem. If the problem is allowed to fester, it can have a damaging effect on the relationship.

If you are concerned about your sex life, you need to voice your concerns to your spouse, not in an accusatory way ("You never want to have sex anymore") but in a nonemotional, matter-of-fact way ("Gee, we don't seem to have time for each other anymore"). Once the problem is aired, you can begin to discuss ways to deal with it.

The first and most important step is for a couple to establish a life that is separate and distinct from the one they have with their children. In order to ensure privacy, past a certain hour of the night, a parent's bedroom should be off limits except in the case of emergencies. I have known some men who actually believed that they were impotent but, in fact, were just victims of constant interruption by children! After a few thwarted efforts at having sex, they simply stopped trying.

There are solutions, but planning is often required. Perhaps on occasion a grandparent can baby-sit overnight on a weekend so that you can get away alone, or perhaps you can arrange to have your children spend the night at a friend's house so you can be alone (and you can reciprocate for them). As long as there is communication between spouses, these problems are not insurmountable. Interestingly, some of my patients seemed to enjoy better sex lives when we discuss their doing a few things to improve their own self-image. A woman who devotes some time to herself inevitably feels more valuable and therefore more attractive. One busy young lawyer I particularly admired profited a great deal from going for a facial and massage once a week and from seeing a nutritionist and exercise trainer to improve her physical condition. The first part of our discussion was devoted to encouraging her to believe she was worth the investment of time and money all this required. The second was planning small interventions she saw first as indulgences but later agreed helped her look and feel better. Her renewed interest in herself seemed to kindle both an expectation of more attention from her husband and an increased appreciation of her by him: She reported a marked step up in the frequency and caliber of their sexual encounters within just a few months of her new regime:

Q. *Can sex aggravate a heart condition?*

A. Like any physical activity, sexual intercourse, particularly when it culminates in orgasm, increases the work of the heart. This does not make it prohibitive, though, and in fact, it can be positively health giving, releasing stress, improving outlook, and lessening the harmful sense of isolation and vulnerability many patients with heart disease experience. I think it important to have careful individual attention from your doctor before resuming sexual activity; some positions are less stressful than others—for example, lying on your back to receive a partner is less stressful than you mounting him and effecting the thrusting, back-and-forth action that creates stimulation. Another issue is to review both the efficacy and side effects of the medications you are taking. If you have a recurrent arrhythmia, it's important to check whether physical activity will make it occur or prolong it when it does. The pain of insufficient blood supply to the heart that may occur when the demand for cardiac work is increased (as in sexual activity) is called angina pectoris. Many patients find that using a coronary dilator like nitroglycerine before sex prevents angina from occurring. Finally, remember that some medications diminish sexual pleasure and even make men less able to have an erection. The chief offenders are often the drugs used to lower blood pressure, and your doctor may have to change the medications you are on so that life returns to a more normal state.

Q. *Is masturbation normal for an adult?*

A. Yes, masturbation is "normal" for adults, especially when there is no significant other or if, for some reason, sexual activity with a partner is suspended. Moreover, in some relationships, one or both partners may be unable to produce orgasm by intercourse alone, and partners routinely climax through masturbation either in the presence of the other or alone later.

Q. *Are there any aphrodisiacs that really work?*

A. Since the dawn of time, men and women have been searching for a magic pill or potion that could enhance sexual interest, potency, and attractiveness. In fact, every big city has a boutique or two offering a wide array of products from body oils to scented candles to herbal formulas—that promise to rev up sexual desire. Are any of these so-called aphrodisiacs effective? There is no scientific evidence that they are. If you are in the mood for sex, a body rub with an exotic oil in a candlelit bedroom may help move things along, but these items are not sexual stimulants. Ironically, camouflaging our natural odors with artificial floral perfume scents may actually have a dampening effect on our sexual partners. Animals (human beings included) are believed to secrete substances through the skin called pheromones that make them attractive to the opposite sex. (The word *pheromone* comes from the Greek words *pherein* to bring or transfer and *hormon* to excite.) Most pheromones are picked up through our sense of smell, although some can be tasted through the skin. Pheromones have been widely studied in animals, but little is known about their role in human behavior. There is always a danger that if we cover up our natural smells with excess lotions and potions, it could actually diminish our sex appeal!

There is one prescription drug available for the treatment of sexual disorders in both men and women: yohimbine (known as yohimbine hydrochloride), a compound extracted from the bark of an African tree. Yohimbine has been shown to successfully treat impotency in some men and can restore the ability to have an erection. The bad news is: Yohimbine can lower blood pressure to dangerous levels and can cause extreme anxiety in some men. There is nothing like a panic attack to reduce libido!

Drugs that affect mood can have very different effects on sexual performance. Prozac, for example, can make it difficult to have an orgasm for both men and women. While a dose of Periactin before you have sex might help— it doesn't always neutralize this unwelcome side effect of Prozac—it is a common reason people discontinue it. Other antidepressants increase libido simply because they lessen sadness; finding the right medication may take more than one try.

Sexual Abuse

Q. *Recently, I had a very upsetting experience. I have been depressed lately and I went to see a therapist who came highly recommended by a friend. After talking to me for less than a half an hour, the therapist suggested that I may have been sexually abused by a parent as a child. I was very shocked by what she said. I have no memory of sexual abuse, and although my relationship with my parents has at times been rocky, I cannot imagine either one of them ever abusing me in that way. Nevertheless, I am deeply disturbed by what the therapist said. I have not returned to her, and really do not know what to do. Should I talk to my parents about this? I am still depressed and am wary of going to another therapist.*

A. I have no doubt that you are confused and shaken by what the therapist told you. I personally have serious doubts about the competency of any mental health professional who would presume to diagnose a patient on the basis of one brief meeting. My advice to you is to proceed with caution.

"Retrieving" memories of sexual abuse is one of the most controversial areas in modern psychiatry. I believe that the usual psychiatric patient is sick, regressed, vulnerable, and suggestible, particularly when the person doing the suggesting is the therapist, often invested by the patient with near magical power and omnipotence. Although it may be possible to repress a bad memory for years and even decades, many psychiatrists are highly skeptical of these claims, and feel that if this phenomenon does occur, it is at best extremely rare.

Although we do not want to regress to the days when therapists dismissed legitimate complaints of sexual abuse as mere fantasy, it can be equally destructive to diagnose sexual abuse when, in fact, it did not occur. I have seen such "retrieved" memories cause irremediable pain for both patient and for the parent, relative, or other individual blamed for the abuse that may be a totally unwarranted assumption by the therapist. Accusing a family member of sexual abuse does not only affect that one family member; its reverberations can be felt throughout the entire family, and sometimes even the entire community. I have seen these accusations quite literally tear families apart, and even if the accuser recants (as sometimes happens) at a later date, the damage has been done.

I want to stress that I am in no way condoning sexual abuse, or suggesting that true abusers should be protected. I am fully aware that in our society, abusers of children are often protected by feelings of denial among the other family members and a community that may be fearful to interfere with the private life of a family. In the situation that you are describing, however, when the victim has no memory of the incident, I feel it is wrong to rely on the word of one therapist who barely knows you. I advise you to see another therapist, preferably one who is recommended by your physician, to help you sort out this matter.

Sexually Transmitted Diseases

Q. *Can you get a sexually transmitted disease by sitting on a public toilet seat?*

A. If an organism that causes a disease can only be passed through sexual contact, such as in the case of chlamydia, gonorrhea, herpes, and syphilis, then you cannot contract the disease by sitting on a toilet seat. There is one type of STD, however, that can be transmitted by contact with an infected toilet seat: pediculosis pubis or crabs. Crabs can be passed by body-to-body contact, but they can also be passed through the use of shared sheets, towels, clothing, and using the same toilet seat as an infected person. These pesky organisms can attach to pubic hair and other hairy parts of the body, and can cause mild to moderate itching. Crabs are easy to diagnose: Although they are small, you can see them and you certainly will feel them. Fortunately, crabs can be eliminated by using any number of medicated shampoos, sold either over-the-counter or by prescription.

Q. *At my last visit to the gynecologist, I was diagnosed with genital warts inside my vagina. Since I did not have any symptoms, I was very surprised to hear that anything was wrong, and, frankly, I do not even know from whom I got them. My doc-*

tor said that in all likelihood the warts would go away, and since I was not in any discomfort, he did not recommend any treatment. He also scared me a little bit by telling me that I must come in every six months for a Pap smear because these warts increase my risk of cervical cancer. How dangerous are these warts? What can I do about them?

A. Known medically as condyloma, sexual warts—small soft bumps in or near the vagina, penis, or rectum—are a virtual epidemic in the United States and are passed from person to person during unprotected sexual intercourse. Genital warts are caused by the human papilloma virus (HPV), which affects as many as 50 million Americans. The warts can surface up to three months after the initial contact. If you have had different sexual partners within a three-month period, you could have been exposed to HPV from any one of them. Genital warts are most common among sexually active young adults between the ages of twenty and twenty-four. Women at high risk of contracting genital warts are those who have had other sexually transmitted diseases, such as herpes or chlamydia; are pregnant; use oral contraceptives; or have compromised immune systems due to other illnesses. Genital warts are usually painless and, quite often, someone with warts may be completely unaware of them. As in your case, they may be detected by an observant doctor, or detected on an abnormal Pap smear. In some cases, the warts may cause some itching and burning or discomfort during sex.

Treatment varies depending on the severity of the problem and the location of the warts. If you only have a few warts and are not experiencing any symptoms, your physician may decide to wait and see if the condition clears up on its own; in about 25 percent of all cases, it will. If you are in great discomfort and the warts are located outside of the vaginal area, your physician may prescribe a medicine to be used externally that dries up the warts, or an acid that burns them off. Internal warts may be frozen off in a procedure called cryosurgery, or burned off with an electric current in a procedure called electrocautery. If the warts are very large, surgical removal may be necessary.

The human papilloma virus has been associated with an increased risk of cervical cancer as well as invasive cancer of the vulva. Your doctor was right in telling you to be vigilant about your Pap tests, which will detect any cancerous changes at the earliest stages when the prognosis for a cure is excellent. I also recommend that you make sure that you get enough folic acid in your diet. Researchers at the University of Alabama recently found that women with the lowest blood levels of folic acid, a B vitamin, were the most likely to develop cervical dysplasia, a precancerous condition. These researchers suggested that folic acid may offer some protection against HPV.

Folic acid can be found in foods such as spinach, asparagus, and wheat germ and in multivitamin supplements. Be sure to get at least 400 mcg. daily of this essential vitamin.

Q. *What is the difference between a fever blister genital herpes? Can herpes spread from the mouth to the genital area during oral sex?*

A. Yes, a fever blister and genital herpes are caused by the same virus, and you can definitely get genital herpes from a lover who has an oral herpes infection. There are two types of herpes virus: HPV I and HPV II. HPV I is usually the cause of oral sores, and HPV II most often strikes the genital (penis, vagina, cervix, thighs) or anal area; however, this is not always the case.

Herpes is usually not serious, but the blisters can be painful. Very often, herpes begins with an itching or burning sensation in the vaginal area that can develop into flulike symptoms including fever, swollen glands, and generalized muscle aches. The initial herpes attack may last for close to two weeks. There is no cure for herpes; once you contract the virus, it can lie dormant after the acute lesion or episode subside. It causes periodic flare-ups that are typically not as severe as the first. Antibiotics are useless against the herpes virus, but the antiviral drug acyclovir (Zovirax) used topically or taken orally can reduce the severity of symptoms. Stress, fatigue, illness, or even the hormonal changes of menopause can trigger a herpes attack. It can also reoccur during pregnancy, and there is a small risk that it can be transmitted to the fetus and cause miscarriage, blindness, and brain damage to the fetus. Any woman with a history of herpes should be closely watched by her obstetrician for signs of a flare-up. If she has an active genital infection at the end of her pregnancy, the mother may require a cesarean delivery to protect her infant from exposure to and infection with the virus.

The real risk with herpes is that it can spread to the eyes and cause blindness. During a herpes flare-up, you must be scrupulous about washing your hands with soap and water before touching your eyes. Herpes has been linked to an increased risk of cervical cancer in women; if you have a history of herpes, you must have a Pap smear every six months to detect any cancerous changes in the cervix. If caught early, this form of cancer is highly treatable. Herpes may also make you more vulnerable to contract other sexually transmitted diseases; therefore, if you have a history of herpes, you must be vigilant about practicing "safe sex."

The use of a condom can prevent the spread of genital herpes (or oral herpes in the case of oral sex). Do not think that you can avoid herpes simply by abstaining from sex with a partner who has obvious sores: Many people with herpes do not have any symptoms at all, yet are carrying the virus. In fact, some 30 million Americans are thought to have the herpes virus, and if you are sexually active outside of a monogamous relationship, the odds of encountering a partner with herpes are good. In order to avoid spreading the infection, it is advisable not to have sex if you or your partner are in the midst of a herpes attack or have a visible blister.

Skin Care

Q. *I'm forty years old and my back has started to break out again like it did when I was a teenager. How does someone my age deal with acne?*

A. Acne typically occurs between the ages of eighteen and twenty-four, but it can reoccur at any age. Acne results from an accumulation of sebum, the fatty substance secreted by the glands of the hair follicles. Male sex hormones, called androgens, which are produced by both sexes, stimulate the production of sebum. This is why acne often strikes during the teenage years, when hormone levels are soaring. Not every skin rash, however, is true acne. Very often, women who work out may develop an acnelike rash that is actually a bacterial infection from friction caused by the accumulation of sweat under tight exercise clothes. The cure for this condition is simple: wear looser clothes during exercise, shower immediately after working out, and dry off completely before getting dressed. In some cases, your doctor may prescribe a topical antibiotic ointment or systemic antibiotics to knock out the infection.

If these simple measures do not solve your problem, then you should see your physician. During middle age, acne in women may be caused by a change in the balance of estrogen and testosterone in their bodies or an increase in the amount of testosterone they produce. If your blood testosterone levels are elevated, your physician may prescribe hormone therapy to normalize your testosterone level, which should help to clear up your skin. Antibiotics and vitamin A cream may also help to wipe out the acne. A dermatologist can remove excess sebum; sometimes he has to make a small incision over the area and then use another instrument that pushes the sebum out of its pocket beneath the surface to the outside. See your dermatologist first: Even an experienced cosmetician can create infections or do an incomplete job on one or more areas.

For severe acne, a physician may prescribe a synthetic form of vitamin A called Accutane. Taken orally for several months, Accutane reduces the production of sebum, thus helping to control acne. Accutane works well and is safe to use; however, it has a potentially devastating side effect: If a woman gets pregnant while taking this medication, it will cause serious birth defects. Therefore, physicians who prescribe Accutane to women of child bearing age insist that their patients use a reliable form of birth control. In fact, dermatologist Harold Mermelstein, an associate professor at New York University Medical School, instructs his female patients on Accutane to use two forms of birth control to prevent any unintended pregnancies. Dr. Mermelstein advises his patients to wait for the completion of at least one normal menstrual cycle after discontinuing the Accutane before getting pregnant.

Q. *I am in my early fifties, and have kept trim and fit. Although I feel wonderful, I think I look older than I should because I used to spend a great deal of time in the sun and, as a result, have more than my share of wrinkles on my face. Short of surgery, what can I do to get rid of these wrinkles? Do face creams help? What about Retin-A and alphahydroxy acids?*

A. In recent years, there has been an explosion in the number of skin care products on the market that claim to erase wrinkles and rejuvenate tired, old skin. The good news is, some of them actually work, at least up to a point. Depending on how aggressive you want to be, and how much money you want to spend, there are a number of products that you can use that will restore a more youthful appearance to older or sun-damaged skin. Although some products are sold over-the-counter, the most effective treatments are available by prescription only, and can be quite costly. Here are some of your options.

Retin-A Retin-A is a form of topical vitamin A that has been approved by the FDA to treat advanced cases of acne. In the 1980s, dermatologists made the surprise discovery that Retin-A not only cleared up acne, but it also appeared to erase fine lines and wrinkles. Although it has not been approved by the FDA for this use, it has not stopped hundreds of thousands of people from using Retin-A as the ultimate "wrinkle cream," and making it one of the most frequently prescribed topical medications. Retin-A has a mild inflammatory effect on the skin that produces swelling and plumps out the skin, thus filling in small wrinkles, at least temporarily. It does not work well on deep-set wrinkles. Manufacturers of Retin-A claim that this cream can increase collagen, the type of tissue that keeps skin tautly stretched and diminishes sagging. Retin-A increases sun sensitivity, and people who use this product must be careful to avoid the sun or they can get badly burned. The effects of Retin-A are short-lived, and once you stop using the product, the wrinkles return. Many women who use Retin-A are very happy with the result. Talk to your doctor about whether Retin-A would work for you.

Alphahydroxy acids Touted as the "hot" and "new" skin care products of the 1990s, versions of alphahydroxy acids (AHAs) have been used since the days of Cleopatra to keep skin soft and supple. AHAs occur naturally in fruits, sugar cane, and yogurt; they include fruit acids, lactic acid, and glycolic acid. Although there are numerous AHAs on the market offered by nearly every major cosmetic company, they all work in basically the same way. All AHAs are exfoliants that peel away the dead cells from the surface of the skin, giving the skin a smoother, less wrinkled appearance. Manufacturers of these products claim that AHAs can work below the surface of the skin, and can cause real biological changes that truly rejuvenate skin. Most of the dermatologists that we talked with, however, feel that there is not enough scientific evidence to substantiate this claim. The experts do agree, however, that in high enough concentrations, alphahydroxy acids can reduce the appearance of fine wrinkles and give the skin a fresher glow. The alphahydroxy products that are sold over-the-counter vary according to acid content: most contain anywhere between 2 and 10 percent pure alphahydroxy acids. Many dermatologists feel that these over-the-counter products are not strong enough to make a real difference in the skin and recommend more potent products that are available by prescription only. If you are not happy with the result you are getting from an over-the-counter product, consult with a dermatologist about using a stronger one. Some people find that AHAs can be irritating; if you develop any irritation discontinue the product. Do not apply AHAs near your eyes.

Patients who are willing to subject themselves to a more aggressive anti-wrinkle treatment may opt for a "light" chemical peel, which is performed by a dermatologist or a plastic surgeon. In this procedure, a much higher concentration of AHAs (up to a 70 percent solution) is used to literally burn off the top layers of skin. (Deeper chemical peels are done with even stronger acids, trichloroacetic acid or phenol.) The patient is usually given a topical anesthetic, and the remaining skin is sore and tender for up to ten days. Although some beauty salons offer chemical peels with relatively high solutions of AHAs, the risk of a severe burn, scarring, or infection is great unless the peel is administered properly. Therefore, chemical peels should only be performed by a dermatologist or plastic surgeon who is experienced in doing this procedure.

Antioxidants The latest entry into the skin-care game are topical creams that include common antioxidants such as vitamins E and C and some more exotic ones (such as compounds derived from algae). The manufacturers of these antioxidant skin-care products purport that they can protect the skin from damage inflicted by free radicals, unstable molecules that can damage DNA and cause premature wrinkling. Do they work any better than AHAs or Retin-A? Only time will tell. These products have not been used long enough to see if they really make a difference. In some cases, consumers are urged to use antioxidant treatments in conjunction with AHAs—especially if the cosmetic company sells both kinds of products. My advice: If you are intrigued by these products, go ahead and try them. But keep in mind that some of them are very pricey. Inexpensive vitamin E creams in less fancy packaging are available at pharmacies and health food stores. They may work as well as these fancier antioxidants and are far kinder to your pocketbook. One word of caution: Some women can develop an allergic reaction to vitamin E. Try testing the cream on a small area of skin on your upper arm and wait twenty-four hours to see if there is an adverse reaction before putting it all over your face or body.

Estrogen replacement therapy Estrogen replacement therapy improves the ability of skin cells to hold water, so skin becomes thicker and retains more moisture. Estrogen may also stimulate the production of the body's natural moisturizing agent, hyaluronic acid.

Wrinkle prevention Here are some tips on how to prevent further wrinkling:

- Most wrinkles are caused by exposure to ultraviolet light. Therefore, the best way to keep your face wrinkle-free is to wear a sunscreen with an SPF of at least 15 under your makeup.
- Avoid cigarettes. Smokers develop telltale "squint" lines around their eyes and mouth.

- Wear sunglasses. Constant squinting can promote wrinkling around the eyes.
- Slather on the moisture cream early and often. Moisture cream can reduce the appearance of fine lines, and if reapplied throughout the day can keep skin younger-looking. You need not spend a fortune on a skin cream; a recent article in *Consumer Reports* rated the cheaper creams higher than some of the more expensive ones.

Q. *I recently saw a report on television about laser surgery for wrinkles. It was truly amazing: The doctor literally zapped away fine lines and crow's-feet in a matter of seconds. Is this for real? Is it safe?*

A. The procedure you are describing is called laser resurfacing, and it is the very latest surgical treatment for the removal of wrinkles. Here's how it works: Laser energy is delivered in thin, short bursts of invisible, high-energy light that literally burns away lines and wrinkles. Lasers can also be used to remove moles, sunspots, and precancerous lesions on the skin.

Roy Geronemus, M.D., director of the Laser and Skin Surgery Center of New York, one of the pioneers in the use of lasers, says that laser resurfacing not only removes wrinkles superficially but appears to strengthen the underlying collagen under the skin, thus producing a younger, tauter skin.

As good as laser resurfacing sounds, there are some important things to consider before signing up. First, it is a relatively new procedure, and critics are quick to point out that there are no long-term studies to determine its safety. This does not mean it is unsafe, but you should be aware of the fact that it is still uncharted territory and the long-term effects are unknown. Second, not every physician with a laser is qualified to use one. There are no criteria or specialty board that can certify that a physician has undergone the necessary training to be a laser surgeon. In the wrong hands, the laser can be very dangerous, and can result in severe burns and permanent scarring. How does a patient find a qualified, skilled laser surgeon? I offer this advice:

- Someone can be an excellent physician, but it does not mean he has the background or experience to work with lasers. Before submitting to laser surgery, ask the physician about his or her experience with lasers. Find out what kind of training he has had to use a laser. Specifically ask, How many of these procedures have you done? The physician should have performed a number of procedures similar to yours. If you need more reassurance, ask to speak to some of his patients.
- Laser resurfacing should only be performed by a dermatologist or a plastic surgeon. It is not enough that someone know how to handle the laser,

that person must also be knowledgeable in postoperative skin care. You do not jump off the operating table with a new face: It can take several weeks for the laser treatment to fully heal, and some patients may require special care. Finally, you need to know that laser resurfacing of the face can be expensive: A full face peel can cost anywhere between $2,000 to $6,000, which is about twice as much as the traditional acid peel. Cosmetic surgery is rarely, if ever, covered by insurance.

Q. I know the sun is dangerous, but what about tanning beds used in salons? Can I get a safe tan indoors?

A. There is no such thing as a safe tan, period. It really does not matter if you get your tan on a Caribbean beach or in a tanning booth at your local tanning salon: Any tan is a sign of injury to the skin. Until recently, it was believed that the sunlamps used in tanning salons were safe because they only emitted the ultraviolet A (UVA) portion of the light spectrum, unlike real sunlight, which includes both UVA and UVB. Today, we know that UVA can be just as harmful as UVB. In fact, according to one Swedish study, people under age thirty who used tanning beds more than ten times a year incurred more than seven times the risk of developing melanoma, a serious form of skin cancer.

My advice: Steer clear of tanning salons.

Swimming Pools and
Health Risks

Q. *My family belongs to a local pool club. I've noticed that every summer when swimming season begins, we all seem to get a lot more colds and viral infections. Can viruses be transmitted in water? I'm not particularly worried about catching a cold or two, but I am concerned about the risk of contracting a more serious virus such as HIV, the one that causes AIDS.*

A. Let me first answer your question by reassuring you that chlorine, which is routinely used to disinfect swimming pools, kills almost all possible agents of infection except for some very rare ones that are not normally found in the United States. HIV, the AIDS virus, is particularly fragile and will not survive in a chlorine-treated pool. In fact, chlorine is such an effective disinfectant that even if someone who is HIV positive accidentally bleeds into a swimming pool, there is virtually no risk that other swimmers will contract the infection through contact with the water.

Your observation is correct, however, that colds can be transmitted more easily in swimming pools, especially among children. The reason has little to do with the wet environment and everything to do with the fact that kids tend to engage in a great deal of horseplay and physical contact in the

208

water, and, thus, spread their cold germs by touching, sneezing, and coughing on each other. Keep in mind that unlike the pesky common cold, HIV
is not spread through so-called casual contact and, therefore, can only be
transmitted in very specific ways, notably through sexual contact or the
exchange of blood.

Although chlorine can kill the AIDS virus under normal circumstances,
the presence of chlorine in the water will not protect you against contracting HIV if you have sexual intercourse with an HIV positive partner in a
swimming pool.

Tattoos and Body Piercing

Q. *My boyfriend wants us to get matching tattoos. I think it's a nice idea, but I'm a little worried about whether there is any health risk. Are tattoos safe?*

A. Before I even deal with the health issue, keep in mind that tattoos are permanent and your relationship may not be. Before you go to all the fuss and expense of getting a tattoo, ask yourself whether this relationship will last…your tattoo certainly will. Permanent tattoos can only be removed surgically, which can be expensive and painful.

As a physician, I must warn you that there are real health risks involved in any procedure involving needles. There is not only a risk of contracting the AIDS virus from a contaminated needle, but the very real and even more likely risk of contracting hepatitis B. Hepatitis is an inflammation of the liver; hepatitis B is a chronic and virulent form of this disease that can be potentially deadly and is on the rise in the United States. Hepatitis B is transmitted primarily through blood, saliva, or semen. Fortunately, there is a vaccination against hepatitis B, and if you are considering getting a tattoo, you and your boyfriend should first be vaccinated against this disease. The vaccine is a rather expensive procedure, costing more than $100, and involves three separate injections over a period of several months. However, since hepatitis B is potentially deadly, it is well worth the cost and inconvenience. When you finally go for the tattoo, be sure to use a reputable tattoo parlor that only uses disposable, sterile needles. Make sure that the tattoo artist opens up a fresh package containing a clean needle for both you and your boyfriend. Don't take his or her word for it that the needle is new: Have the package opened in front of you.

The same goes for body piercing. Lately, I've noticed more and more young women getting various parts of their bodies pierced from their ears to their nose to their genitals. A hepatitis B vaccination is essential before getting any part of your body pierced. Needless to say, be sure the operator uses a sterile, clean needle for piercing. In addition, do not exchange jewelry with friends, because there is also a risk that you could contract an infection from someone with hepatitis B or who is HIV positive.

Tuberculosis

Q. *Recently, I read that a passenger with tuberculosis infected several other passengers on an airplane. Since I'm a frequent flier, I'm worried that I'm putting myself at risk for this disease. If I do get TB, can it be cured? I know there are new strains of TB that are antibiotic resistant.*

A. There is a rise in TB in the United States, which is particularly worrisome because it is a highly contagious disease. You can get TB by simply inhaling air into which an infected person has coughed up the tubercle bacillus. Any situation in which people are crowded together for a significant period of time can promote the spread of the infection. There have been several cases in which patients and physicians have contracted TB in hospitals. As of this writing, there has been one recorded case of tuberculosis transmission from one passenger to other passengers who were sitting nearby on a commercial airline. Although the passengers all tested positive for TB, meaning that they were exposed to the tubercle bacillus, they were not actively sick. In fact, most people exposed to TB will not get sick—the bacteria will remain dormant in the body. Prompt treatment greatly reduces any chances of an infection developing. People who are at greatest risk of contracting TB are those with weakened immune systems, such as AIDS patients, and poor people who live in crowded, substandard conditions. Although the air on airplanes can be very stuffy, it passes through an air filtration system that can filter out TB bacteria. Unless you are sitting close to a person with an active case of TB, and are in a particular risk group, your chance of getting TB on an airplane is extremely slim.

You are quite right that TB is growing resistant to mainstay drugs. At one time, we used to treat TB with three or even two medicines. Today, the doctor has to literally bombard the infected individual with four drugs (isoniazid, rifampin, pyrazinamide, and either ethambutol or streptomycin). For patients who are at very high risk-that is, who have severely compromised immune systems—up to six drugs may be required. After treatment, patients typically become sputum negative within two weeks—that is, there is no sign of the tubercle bacillus in their saliva.

If you are concerned about whether you have been exposed to the bacillus, ask your doctor to give you a simple skin test in which she injects a tiny amount of protein prepared from the tubercle bacillus itself. If you have met the organism before, you will have antibodies that will recognize the skin deposit and make a red, raised lump or series of lumps on the skin within twenty-four to forty-eight hours. If your test is positive and you have never been vaccinated against the tubercle bacillus (a common medical custom in Europe several decades ago; the vaccine was called BCG) and have never been diagnosed with and treated for active infection, you will have to take for at least six months a drug called isoniazid (you'll need 300 mgm. a day) in combination with pyridoxine, one of the B vitamins (50 mgm. once daily). This is to wipe out any trace of an organism that might potentially infect you. Your doctor will test your blood for any signs of liver damage periodically during your course of therapy.

Urinary Incontinence

Q. You know the expression, "I laughed so hard I almost wet my pants?" Well, it's happening to me, and I can tell you that it is nothing to laugh about. I have started to lose urine when I laugh or cough or when I work out at the gym (which I have stopped doing). Even though I wear a sanitary pad all the time '"just in case," I live in fear of having an accident. In fact, I have stopped playing tennis with my friends because I have found that all the running around seems to make it worse. Is there anything I can do to prevent this from happening?

A. Although urinary incontinence is one of the most common problems among women of *all* ages, it is the one that is least talked about. Women do not talk to each other about it, and they certainly are not talking about it with their physicians. In fact, it is estimated that 90 percent of all cases of incontinence may go unreported. Why the silence? For many women, losing bladder control is not merely a physical problem, it is a blow to their self-esteem. It is associated with aging, dependency, and debility; we tend to think that incontinence is a problem of either infancy or very old age. In reality, studies have shown that as many as half of all women have some type of incontinence problem during their lives. Although incontinence often occurs in older women, as many as one third of all premenopausal women may suffer bouts of incontinence. In the "old old" population, incontinence (of either urine or feces or both) is one of the major reasons why otherwise healthy women wind up in nursing homes.

Once incontinence strikes, many women hide themselves away, steering clear of activities that may bring it on. Rather than risk embarrassment, they drop out of exercise classes (which can have a profound impact on their health and well-being), shun the tennis court, and live in fear of having an accident. Many stop having sex because they're afraid they will spill urine after orgasm. Sadly, this can lead to social isolation and, in some cases, marital discord. On the bright side, there are many things that can be done today to help patients deal with incontinence, and there is absolutely no reason why any woman with this problem should have to restrict her activities in any way. Another positive sign is that some women have begun to break the silence; they are setting up support groups for each other and providing information to others on how to handle this problem. (See Resources, page 224.)

Your particular problem sounds like a very common condition called *stress incontinence*, which is defined as the involuntary loss of urine during periods of increased abdominal pressure. In other words, when you cough, bend down, lift a heavy object, or even laugh too hard you may begin to leak urine. Stress incontinence is usually caused by a weakening of the muscles that support the bladder and is very common among women who have had children by normal spontaneous vaginal deliveries. In some cases, stress incontinence may also be due to a prolapsed or dropped uterus, which occurs when the ligaments of the uterus become stretched and no longer hold the uterus in place. As a result, it may press down on the bladder.

There are other forms of incontinence that may be even more annoying. One common type, *urge incontinence*, is the inability to control urination after you feel the need to go. When your body is working well, the bladder fills with urine, which sends a message to the brain that it is time to empty your bladder, giving you time to find a bathroom. Urine travels from the bladder through an opening called the urethra. The flow of urine is controlled by sphincter muscles that we can open and close at will. At the appropriate time, we relax the sphincter muscle, and we pass the urine. But in the case of urge incontinence, the muscles that guard the opening through which urine passes to the outside seem to contract suddenly without warning or without proper control from the brain. In other words, regardless of whether you are ready to urinate, you do. Many women who have stress incontinence may also suffer from urge incontinence.

Incontinence of all types can be caused by many different factors. As we age, the bladder loses some of its ability to stretch, and may not be able to hold the same amount of urine that it once did. As a result, urine may leak out. In addition, the sphincter muscle that controls the urine flow from the bladder may weaken, contract without proper control by the brain, or simply not work as well as it used to, thus allowing urine to spill through. After menopause, when estrogen levels drop, the urethra wall may thin, shorten, and even move out of alignment, thus compromising its ability to prevent urine from flowing to the outside. Hormone replacement therapy or a local estrogen cream can help relieve this problem by, among other things, replenishing the cells lining the urethra.

Simple measures such as watching your intake of certain types fluids may help with incontinence. For example, caffeine is a mild diuretic. I have found that by simply eliminating caffeine, many women have been able to significantly reduce their episodes of incontinence. (This does not only mean passing on coffee, but also reducing your intake of iced tea, colas, and other caffeinated drinks.) Alcohol is also a mild diuretic that is likely to stimulate urination.

Women suffering from any form of incontinence should see their physicians first to determine the cause and second to see what treatment options are available. In very rare cases, incontinence could be a sign of a more serious problem such as a tumor in the bladder or the aftereffects of a stroke, and, therefore, should not be ignored. Incontinence could also be a sign of a urinary tract infection (page 200), which should be treated promptly or it could spread to the kidneys. The following is a review of the latest methods used to treat urinary incontinence.

Do your kegels Many women with stress incontinence find that a simple exercise can help them regain control of their bladders. Known as kegels, these exercises help to strengthen the pelvic floor, thus providing more support for the bladder and the urethra. They are easy to do, and quite effective if done correctly. In a sitting or standing position, simply squeeze your pelvic muscles tightly, hold for a count of five, and slowly release. Repeat up to a hundred times daily. In order for this exercise to be effective, you must use the correct muscle group. There is an easy way to make sure that you are using the right muscles: When you are urinating, squeeze in and hold back the urine stream. The muscles that you need to control the flow of urine are the same muscles that you need to exercise. If you still feel that you're not using the right muscles, your physician can give you some devices that may help. For example, weighted, tamponlike vaginal cones can be inserted in the vagina. In order to keep the cone firmly in place, you must press down on it using the correct muscles. As you get stronger, you can switch to heavier cones. Another device, called a perineometer, is a thin, air-filled cylinder that is inserted into the vagina and is attached to a gauge outside the body. As the woman squeezes her vaginal muscles, the gauge registers the strength of her contractions. The perineometer not only helps you better isolate the appropriate muscles, it lets you monitor your progress.

Medication Many different types of drug therapies have been useful in helping to control incontinence. Drugs such as ephedrine, imipramine, and phenylpropanolamine hydrochloride can help strengthen the action of the sphincter muscles, which may help control stress incontinence. Other classes of drugs have been shown to help overflow and urge incontinence.

Bladder training Researchers at the National Institute on Aging (NIA) recently reported that bladder training based on behavioral modification can help many women learn to control their incontinence. In the program, patients are put on a schedule for urination and are conditioned to gradually increase the intervals between urination. According to the NIA, women who have taken the program can reduce the number of incontinent episodes by as much as 57 percent. This type of treatment is useful for some but not all patients. Similar programs are offered at many hospitals; to locate one in your area, check with the urology department at a local medical school or hospital.

Vaginal devices Devices that can be inserted into the vagina, such as pessaries or specific anti-incontinence devices that support the weakened or sagging anterior vaginal wall, can be used to treat stress incontinence.

Surgery If the incontinence is caused by a defect of the bladder or a prolapsed uterus, surgery can, in some cases, correct the problem. For example, if the bladder is not in the correct position, the surgeon may be able to move it back into its proper place. In the case of a prolapsed (fallen) uterus, it may be possible to move the uterus back into place so that it is no longer pressing down on the bladder.

Electrical stimulation therapy A new electrical stimulation device produced significant improvement of pelvic muscle strength and reduced the severity of stress incontinence in 40—90 percent of treated patients. The device is made of silicone rubber with carbon electrodes and is used twice a day for fifteen minutes the first four weeks and thirty minutes for the remainder of the twelve-week program. Ask your urologist or gynecologist where to get this newer type of therapy.

Collagen injections In some cases, injections of collagen in the urethra can reduce the size of the opening of the urethra, thus helping to tighten the sphincter muscle. This procedure, which can be done under a local anesthetic, may be useful for women with stress incontinence due to sphincter deficiency.

Estrogen replacement therapy ERT can correct urinary tract incontinence in some patients. It can also diminish the frequency of urinary tract infections when the patient's vulnerability is at least in part the consequence of a thinned, weakened urethral lining.

Q. *Much to my embarrassment, since my husband died, I have been wetting my bed at night. Why is this happening and what can I do to stop it?*

A. I have had several adult patients who are otherwise functioning perfectly well, but who, after a trauma such as the death of a spouse or divorce, have had one or more episodes of wetting the bed. They are often ashamed and bewildered by what they believe is a sign of infantile or regressive behavior. In reality, they are experiencing a normal, physical reaction to stress that happens to many, many people. At night, our bodies produce an antidiuretic hormone that inhibits urination so that we can sleep for hours on end undisturbed. When people are under acute stress, however, this hormone may not be secreted normally, which may cause them to urinate in their sleep. Once the stressful period passes, the problem disappears. Repeated bed wetting by an adult needs a physician's attention to determine its cause. If the condition persists, your doctor needs to evaluate you.

Urinary Tract Infections

Q. *I have a new boyfriend, but right after we started having sex I developed a bladder infection that keeps coming back even after I take antibiotics. Needless to say, this has put a damper on my sex life. What can I do to keep these infections at bay?*

A.Next to the common cold, bladder infections (also known as cystitis) are probably the most common malady to afflict women. In fact, it has been estimated that as many as 20 percent of all women will sometime during their lives suffer from cystitis or some other infection of the urinary tract (which includes the bladder and kidneys), and 90 percent of those who get this problem will have a recurring episode.

The symptoms of urinary tract infections (UTIs) can be very annoying, and include frequent urination (sometimes up to fifty or sixty times a day) or the constant feeling that you have to urinate although you pass very little urine, burning during urination, pelvic or abdominal pain, and blood or pus in the urine. In some cases, a mild infection, if untreated, can move up the urinary tract into the kidneys. Fever, chills, dizziness, nausea, vomiting, and other more severe symptoms may indicate the infection has spread. If you experience any of these symptoms, you must call your doctor.

In order to know how to protect yourself against UTIs, you need to understand a bit about why women are so vulnerable to this problem. Although men also get bladder infections, women get them twenty-five times more often, and the reason why women are so susceptible is due in large part to the female anatomy. Urine travels from the kidneys through tubes called the ureters to the bladder. When the bladder is full enough to stimulate the urge to urinate, the urine then passes through a small passageway called the urethra, which leads into the opening in the vagina where the urine is excreted. In women, the urethra is significantly shorter and wider than it is in men, which can cause several problems: First, due to its shape, the female urethra is easily stretched (such as during intercourse), which can cause irritation. Second, unlike the male urethra, which is encased in the protective covering of the penis, the female urethra is very close to both the outside of the body and to the anal area, and thus is more likely to come in contact with bacteria and other contaminants. Third, after menopause, women are at even greater risk of developing UTIs because, as estrogen levels drop, the urethral wall becomes thinner, which makes it more vulnerable to irritation and infection. (Estrogen, in the form of a cream applied externally into the vagina or taken orally, has been shown to help prevent the thinning of the urethral lining in postmenopausal women.) Most urinary tract infections (about 80 percent) are caused by the E. coli bacteria, which typically migrate from the anal area and reach the urethra. A minority of infections may be caused by other organisms, including staphylococcus, chlamydia, and mycoplasma—the latter two are sexually transmitted. In some cases, women may experience symptoms without bacterial infection, which are most likely due to an irritation of the urethra, as in the case of so-called honeymoon cystitis, a condition caused by the irritation of the urethra due to a sudden increase in sexual activity. Activities such as horseback riding or bicycle riding can also irritate the urethra.

During pregnancy, women are also more prone to develop UTI as the fetus grows and pushes down on the bladder, making it difficult to fully empty the bladder, which can promote infection. UTI can cause kidney infection and the resulting high fever and bacterial toxins can even produce a miscarriage during pregnancy. It should be treated promptly.

Treatment In the past, physicians used to routinely culture urine—that is, check for evidence of bacterial infection and for the particular type of organism—before dispensing antibiotics. Today, in most cases, as soon as a woman shows the telltale symptoms of UTI, her physician will usually prescribe a short course of broad spectrum antibiotics that are effective against many different types of bacteria. The drugs most often used to treat UTIs are sold under the names of Bactrim, Septra, or Cipro. Usually a short dose of antibiotics, sometimes as short as three days, is enough to clear up the infection. At one time, physicians used to prescribe these medications for much longer periods of time; however, the longer a patient was on an antibiotic, the greater her risk of developing a yeast infection, which may make her more vulnerable to UTIs. Lowering the amount of time you are exposed to antibiotics appears to reduce the risk of developing a yeast infection. In rare cases, however, a woman may have to stay on low levels of antibiotics for a much longer period of time—perhaps several months—and, in some cases, may need to try several different antibiotics in order to find the one that is effective against a particular infection. Women with frequent infections can be given a supply of antibiotics for self-administration when symptoms recur. In most cases, a family doctor, internist, or gynecologist is completely capable of treating a UTI. If a UTI is very persistent, however, the patient should be referred to an urologist.

If you are very sick from a UTI—that is, are vomiting, running a fever, and having severe back pain radiating into your abdomen and groin—you may have to be hospitalized and put on an IV to deliver the medication (which you may not be able to keep down otherwise) and prevent excess fluid loss. In this era of hospitalizing patients less and for shorter and shorter periods of time, though, the treatment is shifting and many patients are now treated with oral antibiotics at home.

Over-the-counter analgesics such as acetaminophen or Motrin can be taken to control pain. If the pain is severe, however, a physician may prescribe antispasmodic drugs, to relax the bladder muscles, or administer a local anesthetic. Although many women find that soaking in a tub of comfortably warm water (if it is too hot, it can irritate the urethra) helps to relieve symptoms, others find this to be irritating. You may have to see what works for you. Some women find that using a heating pad on their abdomen also helps to relieve pain.

Prevention Once a woman develops a UTI, she is at even greater risk of having a recurrence. In many cases, though, UTI can be prevented. Here is some advice on how to control UTI.

Good hygiene Simple measures, such as maintaining a high level of personal cleanliness, can make a big difference in preventing future infections. Keep your genital area clean. After a bowel movement, always wipe from front to back (away from the vagina) so that you do not inadvertently spread bacteria from the anal area to the vaginal and urinary tract openings. Wash your genital and rectal area daily with a nonirritating soap or cleanser. Avoid bubble baths or oils, vaginal deodorant sprays or anything else that may be irritating. Do not share towels with anyone else in your home—it is a good way to pass bacteria back and forth. If you use sanitary pads during menstruation, change them several times a day. The blood that collects on the pads provide a wonderful breeding ground for bacteria, and an easy route for bacteria to travel from one site to another.

Urinate when you need to When you have to urinate, do not ignore the urge; go to the bathroom. If urine is allowed to collect in the bladder, it can promote infection.

Sexual practices Be sure to urinate before and after having sex. Keeping the bladder full during intercourse can be very irritating, and holding in urine afterward can allow any newly introduced bacteria to multiply in the bladder. Make sure that your partner washes his genitals before having sex. If you engage in anal sex, be sure that your partner wears a condom and that he removes the condom and washes before penetrating your vagina.

If you find that you have frequent UTI flare-ups after sexual activity, be careful about doing anything irritating during sex. For example, for many women, the upper position can put too much pressure on the urethra; if this is the case, simply try a position that will be less irritating. In addition, constant stimulation to the clitoral area might also be irritating to the urethra, so try to avoid any activity that will put undue pressure on the clitoral area for an extended period of time.

Some contraceptives may also promote UTI, or aggravate an existing condition. In the past, women on higher-dose birth control pills were at greater risk of UTI; however, today's lower-dose pills appear to be safer in this regard. Barrier methods of contraception may also be problematic for some women. For example, a poorly fitted diaphragm can press against the urethra, thus causing irritation, or the spermicidal jelly that is normally used with the diaphragm can also kill some of the "good" bacteria in the vagina that protects against disease, thus allowing the "bad" bacteria to proliferate. Some women find latex condoms to be quite irritating and, if this is the case, may have to ask their partners to use a different type of condom. (Keep in mind that only latex condoms provide protection against sexually transmitted diseases.) If you have chronic UTI, it is probably a good idea to consult with your doctor about finding the right contraceptive for you.

In some cases, if a woman finds that she frequently has a flare-up after sex, her physician may advise her to take one antibiotic pill prophylactically before intercourse, which may help to prevent infection. In particular, this may be effective in the case of a woman who has not yet grown resistant to the bacteria carried by a new sexual partner.

Eat and drink the right stuff Drink at least eight glasses of water daily. Limit your intake of alcohol or caffeinated beverages, which can irritate the bladder. Avoid the excess intake of sugary foods and refined carbohydrates that may promote the growth of bacteria.

Home remedies As far as I'm concerned, as long as you have consulted with a doctor, there is nothing wrong with trying home remedies, particularly if your goal is to prevent a recurrent infection. I do not recommend, however, that home remedies should be clone to the exclusion of conventional medical treatment. In the case of UTI, some women need all the help they can get to control infection, and all worthwhile treatments—whether they are conventional or not—should be considered.

There are two schools of thought on the self-treatment of UTIs: They are divided into the cranberry faction, and the acid-free faction. Before you can choose sides, you need to understand where and how the battle lines have been drawn.

The cranberry cure For decades, natural healers have prescribed cranberry juice and capsules (which are sold in health food stores) as a traditional remedy for UTI. The medical community scorned this home remedy until recent studies showed that cranberries and blueberries contain compounds that prevent bacteria from building up in the bladder. Thus, the bacteria that can cause infection are flushed out in the urine. Today, countless women drink cranberry juice by the gallon, mash whole cranberries into yogurt, and pop handfuls of cranberry pills (often along with 1,000 mg. of vitamin C daily) when they feel the first sign of a UTI, and many swear that this is all it takes to keep infections at bay.

The acid-free cure On the other hand, some women find that the "cranberry cure" not only does not work for them but, in fact, aggravates their symptoms by increasing the acid content in their urine, which may cause it to burn when it passes through the urethra. At the first sign of infection, these women find relief from the burning during urination by using commercial antacids (such as Tums or Rolaids) to deacidify their urine. Only trial and error will tell which if either of these home remedies will work for you.

Some women find that herbal teas help to prevent infection and reduce symptoms. There are no scientific studies to back up this assertion, but women often recommend teas made from the herb urva usi, a folk remedy used for bladder and kidney ailments that is sold in health food stores.

Vaginal Deodorants

Q. *Should women use vaginal deodorants?*

A. Absolutely not. If you have a bad vaginal odor or discharge, you should not use a deodorant to cover it up. Go to your gynecologist to make sure that you don't have an infection. Normal hygiene bathing or showering daily—should be all you need to prevent unpleasant body odor.

Although we are obsessed with cleanliness and smelling good, normal body odor is not offensive. In fact, animals (humans included) produce scents called pheromones that may be instruments for attracting the opposite sex and causing sexual arousal in partners. Overpowering your natural scent with an artificial fragrance may actually be detrimental to your ability to attract members of the opposite sex!

Finally, many women find vaginal deodorants to be very irritating, and may cause itching and other types of unpleasant side effects.

Vaginal Dryness

Q. I suffer from terrible vaginal dryness that makes intercourse very uncomfortable. What can be causing this problem and, more important, what can I do about it?

A. Vaginal dryness is one of the most common complaints that I hear from women of all ages. Under normal conditions, glands on the cervix produce a discharge that moistens and lubricates the vagina. If these glands do not function properly, the vagina can feel tight and dry. The friction that results from intercourse can be quite irritating. For some women, the monthly fluctuations in estrogen can result in periods of vaginal dryness, especially after their menstrual periods. Similarly, after the postmenopausal drop in estrogen, the production of discharge is diminished, which can cause great discomfort. The drop in estrogen produces other undesirable changes in the vagina, including the thinning of vaginal walls and a loss of its tone and elasticity. This is not only uncomfortable but, in combination with the loss of lubrication, can actually increase the risk of developing an infection, such as candida albicans (yeast), which will only add to your misery.

Vaginal dryness may also be caused by any number of medications, including antihistamines, which in addition to drying out your nose could dry out the mucous lining of the vagina. This is true even of some antidepressants. If you are taking any medications that could contribute to vaginal dryness, check with your physician to see if she can prescribe something different. If you have other symptoms including dry eye and joint pain, vaginal dryness could be a sign of an autoimmune disease such as rheumatoid arthritis. In some cases, vaginal dryness could be caused by an infection, which may also be accompanied by itching and a discharge. You and your doctor need to determine the cause of your discomfort.

There are several steps that you can take to relieve your symptoms. In your local drugstore, you will find a wide variety of vaginal moisturizing creams such as Replens and Gyne-Moistrin. Sold in premeasured, disposable packets, these creams can be inserted in much the same way you would use a tampon. In most cases, women find relief by simply using the cream every other day. If sex is painful, perhaps you need a longer period of foreplay prior to intercourse to help "prepare" the vagina for intercourse. In addition to pro-longing foreplay, you can try using an over-the-counter lubricant such as K-Y Jelly during sex to help reduce friction and make intercourse more enjoyable. You can rub the lubricant on your partner's penis, or topically on your vagina. (Do not use petroleum jelly. It can promote infection by provid-ing a favorable growth environment for yeast and bacteria.)

For postmenopausal women, hormone replacement therapy can have a remarkably rejuvenating effect on the vagina, improving lubrication and strengthening the vaginal lining. If you do not want to take hormones, how-ever, you can try other things. First, I would recommend using an estrogen cream topically in the vagina, which can help reduce many of the unpleas-ant symptoms associated with vaginal dryness. When the cream is used externally, or placed no farther than the length of your index finger's first joint into the vaginal opening, the es trogen is not absorbed by the blood-stream to any significant degree, and should cause no adverse side effects. Over-the-counter vaginal moisturizing creams may help, but they're not as effective as estrogen creams.

Several women have told me that herbal remedies, such as evening prim-rose oil, which is sold in health food stores, can also be quite helpful. Evening primrose oil is sold in capsule form and can be taken orally. Although evening primrose oil has not been clinically tested in a scientific setting for this purpose, many women swear by it.

Varicose Veins

Q. *I hate wearing shorts in the summer because I have ugly varicose veins. They also hurt! What's the best way to get rid of them?*

A. Varicose veins are not only unsightly and in some cases painful, but they can also be dangerous. Varicosities come from a weakness in the wall of the vein, or in the tiny valves that prevent blood from flowing in the wrong direction as it travels up from the legs back to the heart. The veins enlarge, become painful, and, in advanced cases, can allow fluid to leak from the veins out into the tissues so that the ankles and legs become swollen, particularly after periods of prolonged standing.

Varicosities can either be in the venous system that is close to the skin (superficial) or in the deeper veins of the legs. Since the damaged vein wall can cause the formation of blood clots (called thromboses), varicose veins are not simply a cosmetic problem. While a venous thrombosis in the superficial system can usually be treated with leg elevation and warm soaks, clots in the deep venous system are more serious. When these deep clots extend above the knee, they need to be treated with blood thinning medication.

The symptoms of varicose veins include:

- Unsightly dilated, tortuous blue-colored blood vessels in the legs.
- A sensation of pressure, heaviness, or even a dull ache in the legs after standing for long periods of time.
- Swelling of the ankles and legs.
- Ulceration of the skin over the varicose veins because of blood pooling in the area.

The treatment for varicose veins varies depending on the severity of the problem. In milder cases, frequent elevation of the legs and the avoidance of long periods of standing can help to keep symptoms under control. Elastic or "support" hose can also help to avoid leg and ankle swelling. Although many brands of support hose are sold over-the-counter, I recommend that patients see a vascular specialist to have their support hose expertly measured and designed specifically for them. Individually tailored products fit better, are more comfortable, and provide better support.

In more severe cases, your physician will refer you to a competent vascular surgeon for a consultation. In some cases, the surgeon may decide to perform a procedure called sclerotherapy in which she injects into the veins a solution that permanently occludes it and then applies a compression bandage to the site. Within a short time, the vein disappears. Stripping, or actually removing the troublesome vein, is another surgical option that eliminates the problem. The downside with this procedure, however, is some women may be left with a series of small, unsightly scars. You and your surgeon will decide which procedure will work best for your particular situation.

Weight and Health

Q. *I am forty-five years old and have spent at least half my life struggling to keep my weight down. I remember starving myself as a teenager (I once got so thin that my period disappeared for a year!) and going from one fad diet to another throughout my twenties and thirties, bouncing back and forth from a size 5 to a size 12. In recent years, I have finally come to accept that I will not be as thin as a model and have begun to make peace with my 5-foot-5, 145-pound body. I exercise, eat sensibly, and am in pretty good shape. I was chagrined to learn, however, that according to the latest studies, my weight may pose a serious risk to my health. Is this true?*

A. The latest information on weight is based on a comprehensive study that tracked the lifestyle and health of 115,000 registered nurses over a sixteen-year period. The study made headlines with its controversial finding that even a moderate weight gain (more than twenty-two pounds) after age eighteen can greatly increase the risk of early death. Up until this study, it was commonly believed that weight gain was a natural—even inevitable—part of growing older. In fact, the standard weight guideline charts used by insurance companies allowed for a twenty-pound weight gain during adulthood and even had a separate chart for people over thirty-five. Newly revised weight

229

charts have not only downsized the range of permissible weight (by up to eighteen pounds) but no longer base recommendations on age. In other words, what is good for an eighteen-year-old is good for an eighty-year-old.

What was even more surprising about the Nurses' Study was the unexpected finding that the thinnest women were actually the healthiest. Up until this study, it was widely believed that underweight women had the highest mortality rate. On closer examination, however, researchers found that thinness per se was not dangerous, but that many thin women smoked (which greatly increased their risk of succumbing to many different diseases) or were thin as a result of a wasting illness. In reality, according to this study, healthy, thin nonsmokers are actually at the lowest risk of cancer and heart disease than any other group, and destined to live the longest. Despite the fact that thin appears to be better, this does not mean that you need to go on a crash diet. The relationship between weight and health is a complicated one, and cannot be determined simply by reading numbers on a chart; there are many other factors to consider, including body type and lifestyle.

Know your BMI (body mass index) The body mass index calculates weight in proportion to height. It is a useful measurement because it provides some sense of your real risk of dying young or developing a serious disease. Here is how to calculate your BMI. Multiply your weight by 0.45 to get the measure in kilograms. Then, measure your height in inches and multiply that number by 0.0254 to convert to meters. Multiply that number by itself. Divide the result into your weight in kilograms. For example, a 5-foot-5, 145-pound woman like yourself would have a BMI of 24. Based on the Nurses' Study, a BMI of:

19 or less puts you at the lowest risk of early death
19-24.9 raises the risk by 20 percent
27-28.9 raises the risk by 60 percent
29-31.9 raises the risk by 110 percent
more than 32 raises the risk by 120 percent

So what do these numbers mean? Since the risk of early death is very slim to begin with, a 20 percent increase in risk is not very significant. In fact, although the health risks creep up with every pound, the women who are truly at risk are those who are obese, as defined as 30 percent above their desired body weight. Women who are seriously overweight need to seek medical attention to help them reduce.

Most women, however, fall somewhere in between the thinnest and the obese. They may comply with the weight guidelines, but their BMI is in the higher risk range. Should women who may have a few extra pounds to shed lose weight to achieve the lowest risk rating? It all depends.

Yes, if you have other risk factors If you are diabetic, have heart disease, or are at greater risk of getting breast cancer due to family history, you should try to slim down to the lowest risk group that you can tolerate.

Yes, if you have poor health habits If you have terrible health habits—that is, you are eating a high-fat, fast-food diet that is packed with calories and devoid of fiber and nutrients, and rarely, if ever, exercise—it is definitely time for a change in eating style. Switching to a diet low in fat and high in fiber will help shed pounds. If you add regular exercise to your regimen, the pounds will burn off even faster. If you are already eating a sensible diet and getting enough exercise, dieting may be more a bother than it's worth. Numerous studies have shown that most diets simply do not work and that dieters often regain even more weight when the diet is over. In addition, not every woman can diet in a safe, healthy manner.

No, if dieting can become an obsession In an attempt to be thin, some women will fast for days, vomit, exercise excessively, or use laxatives to control their weight. For these women, the abuse to which they are exposing their bodies far outweighs any potential gain from taking off a few extra pounds. There is such a thing as being too thin. Any diet that interrupts the menstrual cycle and other normal bodily functions is dangerous.

Yes, if you have midline obesity Where that extra weight is accumulating is another factor to consider in the decision of whether you need to lose weight. Many studies have shown that women who are shaped more like apples than pears—that is, who have extra fat around their waistline—are at significantly higher risk of having a heart attack than women who carry their weight at their hips and thighs. If you are carrying your extra weight around your waist, you should lose weight *and* combine your reducing diet with exercise to encourage a better distribution of body fat.

Although I do not recommend that everyone who is slightly overweight should go on a strict diet, I do believe that it is desirable to try to maintain normal weight. There is such compelling evidence that being thin is associated with a longer, healthier life that, in this case, prevention really is the best medicine. Women should be careful not to allow those extra pounds to accumulate with each passing year. One way to prevent unwanted weight gain is to be aware of the times in your life when you are most vulnerable to weight gain. For instance, with each pregnancy, the average woman retains seven pounds that she never sheds. The years immediately following menopause are another time in which women typically gain weight. Increased physical activity during these vulnerable periods combined with a well-planned eating program can help prevent unwanted "weight creep."

231

Workplace Health

Q. *I am a secretary for the managing partner of a major law firm. I'm very good at what I do: I spend about six hours a day in front of a word processor typing documents that must be done quickly and accurately. I love my job, but by the end of the day, my neck is killing me and my back feels stiff. Lately, I have been developing shooting pains down both of my arms and my hands sometimes feel numb. I'm very worried that I will have to quit my job. Is there anything I can do to get rid of the pain?*

A. I have seen many women who complain of similar symptoms and who come to my office in dire fear that they will lose their jobs and their means of earning a living. This problem is so commonplace that we have a name for it: repetitive stress injury (RSI). As its name implies, this kind of injury can be caused by any continual, repetitive motion that places undue stress on overused muscles and tendons. Usually the damage is worst in the fingers, hands, arms, and shoulders, but it can affect any part of the body exposed to repeated mechanical stress. Musicians, typists, and computer operators are among those most commonly affected by RSI.

Since the industrial revolution, repetitive stress injury has become a widespread problem. In the past, typical victims were assembly-line workers who

232

drove the same screw into the same nut over and over again, hundreds of times a day. Occasionally, a doctor would see a musician who wore herself down with excessive practicing. Today, however, physicians like myself are treating a new kind of RSI victim: It is becoming increasingly more common to see white-collar office workers with RSI, largely due to the widespread use of computers and word processors. There are some differences between computer keyboards and traditional typewriters that make computer users more prone to RSI. For one thing, computer keyboards do not have carriages that need to be moved at the end of a line, nor do they require breaks at the end of a page to insert a new piece of paper—computer operators can sit for hours typing away and never have to stop and change position. Another virtue of the old-fashioned typewriter was that the keys had to be pushed down and then needed time to spring back into position: Even the fastest typists were limited by this mechanical feature of the machine. Computer keyboards can tolerate much faster typing speeds; the operator can perform many more of the damaging movements in any given time period! All of this may be good for productivity, but it is not good for workers' health. Continually working in a strained position can inflict even more damage if the worker is under a great deal of stress and her muscles are tight and strained and, consequently, easy to fatigue.

Repetitive stress injuries can affect both sexes, but they seem to strike women in greater numbers. One obvious reason is that secretarial pools are mainly female, but anatomical differences between men and women may be another reason. Women tend to have weaker upper-body strength than men and, in particular, weaker wrists. In fact, one kind of repetitive stress injury to the wrist, called carpal tunnel syndrome, is two to six times more likely to strike women than men.

Treatment for repetitive stress injuries varies according to the problem. The overwhelming majority of cases are caused by the deadly combination of poorly designed workplaces and workers who have developed poor keyboard work habits. In most cases, an exercise rehabilitation program and retraining to use a keyboard correctly will solve the problem. In rare cases, surgery may be required, and in even rarer cases, a person may actually have to change occupations. The good news is, most repetitive stress injuries can be prevented, and even if you are currently experiencing problems, there are many things you can do to eliminate the pain and avoid further injury.

Know the symptoms People with RSI often make the mistake of ignoring the early symptoms. It is imperative that people who work in jobs where they are vulnerable to this problem become aware of the early warning signs so they can get prompt medical attention. Here are some of the typical warning signs of RSI:

Pain In the very early stages, you may only feel pain when you stop work, but as the injury worsens, you will feel pain during the task that is giving you trouble. After a while, even some of the simple tasks of everyday living for which you use the same muscles as those you use at work may become more and more difficult. For example, if you are a computer operator, slicing bread or buttoning your clothes may become painful.

Peculiar sensations Many patients begin to complain about strange feelings in the parts of their body that are used over and over, such as numbness and tingling in their hands or arms.

If you are experiencing any of these symptoms, you should seek prompt medical attention.

Finding the right doctor When I see a patient who has a repetitive stress injury, I often refer her to Dr. Emil Pascarelli, founder of the Miller Institute at St. Luke's—Roosevelt Hospital Center in New York, one of the world's foremost centers in the treatment of these problems. Dr. Pascarelli has written the authoritative book on the subject of RSI and currently practices at the Columbia Presbyterian Eastside facility in New York. He is world famous and deservedly so: He has even modified musical instruments for artists to correct harmful positions or damaging movements. Physicians who routinely work with RSI have special training in pinpointing which muscles, bones, and joints are injured and, more important, in devising a treatment plan. There are occupational health centers, where these specialists can be found, throughout the United States. To locate one in your area, call your local medical society.

Redesigning your workplace There are many products on the market today—from keyboards to office chairs—that claim to be "ergonomically designed," meaning that they are designed to avoid injury. The problem is, there is no official, medically approved standard for ergonomic design; literally anyone can claim that a product will reduce injury. Before you invest in any equipment, I suggest you check with a physician who is knowledgeable in RSI. Regardless of what equipment you may use, the same rules apply: You will need to make sure that your seat and desk are designed in such a way so that your body is positioned as naturally as possible. Here are some things to watch out for:

• Make sure that your desk or worktable is the right height. The center of the keyboard should be approximately elbow level when you are seated (between twenty-seven and thirty-five inches above the floor).

• When you are working, your head should be directly over your shoulders, and the monitor should be at eye level, or slightly lower, so that you can maintain the natural curve of your neck as you type. You should sit about an arm's length away from the screen.

- Never set the monitor off to one side so that you need to continually twist your neck in an unnatural and uncomfortable position.
- Find a comfortable chair that provides good upper-body support; this should eliminate those end-of-the-day neck and back aches.
- Your feet should rest comfortably on the floor. Use a footstool to take tension off your lower back; this is a boon for those of us who spend a lot of our lives desk-bound.

The right position Your desk should be arranged so that your elbows and wrists are in a straight line when you work. You must keep your wrists straight when you type: Do not rest them on the keyboard. When your wrists are bent (either upward or downward), you need more force from the muscles in your forearm to move your fingers, which increases the friction on the tendons in the fingers as they move back and forth across the angled wrist. This can cause terrible strain on your wrists and hands.

Check your vision Very often, the glasses that we use for reading may not be the right glasses to use to see the computer screen. Craning to see the computer as you copy data from the printed page can lead to injury. If you find that you are having difficulty seeing, check with your ophthalmologist. Your doctor can make you combination lenses so that you can see both the printed page and the screen equally well with a tiny repositioning of your head. In addition, the work area should be well lit to prevent eyestrain.

Take frequent breaks Every twenty minutes, get up from your desk and stretch your muscles. Take two or three minutes to do some gentle exercises: Slowly move your neck from side to side, do shoulder circles, and loosen your upper body.

Get regular exercise Maintaining good muscle strength will help maintain good posture and strong muscles, which are less likely to be prone to injury.

RSI costs millions of dollars in lost work hours and medical bills each year. It is well worth the effort on the part of both employers and employees to make what are often simple modifications in the workplace that can have a profound impact on worker health and safety.

Q. I frequently come home from work with a headache, and I always seem to have a cold and my eyes are itchy. Many of my co-workers are also constantly sick, and complain of headaches and fatigue. I work in a new high-rise office building where the windows do not open and the air is either too cold or too hot or too stuffy. I used to blame the poor air on the cigarette smokers, but it persisted even after smoking was banned at our office last year. I recently read an article about "sick building syndrome," which said that some offices are breeding grounds for disease! Is this true? Could I be working in one?

A. It certainly sounds as if you could be. Although public concerns over the environment have focused on the problems of outdoor air quality, in reality, indoor air pollution is a growing and perhaps even more serious problem. Studies have shown that the concentration of pollutants in the air are often far worse indoors in many offices and workplaces than outdoors! Indoor pollution is not a minor problem; according to the U.S. Office of Safety and Health Administration (OSHA), as many as 30 percent of all office workers may be exposed to poor air quality at the workplace.

Indoor pollution can be caused by many things, from fumes emitted by chemical cleansers and formaldehyde fumes seeping from new carpet and office furniture to contaminants in the heating, air-conditioning, or ventilating system. Poor ventilation is almost always a culprit. In 1974, in response to the energy crisis precipitated by the Arab oil embargo, building codes were altered to reduce fresh-air ventilation and to improve insulation. Although these changes may have saved countless numbers of barrels of oil, they also drastically reduced the flow of air in and out of many office buildings. To compound the problem, these high-tech, super-sealed, insulated buildings require regular maintenance to keep the air supply fresh, and many building owners are unwilling to pay to adequately maintain their properties. As a result, many buildings are not properly maintained, and employees such as yourself are suffering. In fact, indoor pollution has been linked to many health problems, including headaches, fatigue, dry skin, throat irritation, asthma, sinus problems, and even some forms of cancer. Although there are no national indoor air pollution standards, many localities have regulations of their own. Very often, however, buildings are not inspected for problems unless it is in response to a specific complaint. Therefore, it is up to individuals like yourself to make sure that the air in your workplace is as clean as possible. You and a group of your co-workers should discuss your concerns with your employer and building management. It may also be helpful to contact your local health department or environmental protection agency to come check out the office for potential problems.

Here are some things you can do on your own to minimize your exposure to potentially irritating contaminants:

• Check to see if there is anything in your immediate work area that could be contributing to your problem. For example, do you work near a particular piece of equipment, such as a photocopier, that could be giving off irritating fumes? If you do, perhaps you can have the machine moved to a different part of the office or have your desk moved away from the machine.

• Is there a leak in a pipe or air-conditioning vent that is causing water to accumulate on the ceiling, walls, or carpet? If you see any signs of water, alert building maintenance. Any site where moisture is allowed to collect is a breeding ground for mold, which can be very irritating to many people.

• Ask the building maintenance department to check whether the air-conditioning and heating ducts are working properly. Even if your office gets very cold, I do not advise closing an air-conditioning duct—it will rob you of precious fresh air. A better approach is to ask to have the air redirected so that it is not blowing down on you. In addition, the air-conditioning and heating ducts should be cleaned on a regular basis to avoid accumulation of dust and mold.

Yeast Infections

Q. *For the past few years, I have suffered from constant yeast infections. I have tried just about every over-the-counter preparation and nothing helps. Recently, I read about a pill that is supposed to cure these infections. Will this work? What else can I do?*

A. Yeast infections are probably *the* most common of all gynecological problems; some studies suggest that as many as 75 percent of all women will experience a vaginal yeast infection sometime in their lives. The most common symptoms of a yeast infection are vaginal itching usually accompanied by a thick, white discharge.

There are literally hundreds of different kinds of yeasts (which are actually a type of fungus), but most yeast infections are caused by an overgrowth of candida albicans, a microorganism that is normally found in the vagina. A problem develops when the vagina's natural flora is thrown out of whack, thus allowing the unfettered proliferation of candida.

Many different things can trigger a yeast infection; antibiotics are a common cause because they wipe out the "good" bacteria in the vagina that can keep yeast growth under control. A diet high in sugar, a weakened immune system, oral contraceptives, and extreme stress are all conditions that can

238

make a woman prone to yeast infections. Women who are HIV positive are particularly vulnerable to chronic yeast infections; any woman who is at risk for HIV and has incurable yeast infections should be tested for HIV.

In recent years, many antiyeast medications (mostly topical vaginal creams or suppositories) that were once available by prescription are now available over-the-counter, such as Monistat and Gyne-Lotrimin. (It is important to see your doctor to get an accurate diagnosis before self-prescribing one of these medications—you could have another, more serious type of infection and not know it.) For most women, if used properly, over-the-counter medication will wipe out the infection. There is a group of women, however, for whom these over-the-counter medications are ineffective and stronger prescription medication may be required. If over-the-counter medications do not control your symptoms, check with your doctor about using other types of drugs. A stronger-strength cream or suppository may do the trick. In some cases, it may be necessary to use a stronger cream for a longer period of time, sometimes for weeks or even months. There are some oral antifungal drugs that may work; however, they have unpleasant side effects, including nausea and headaches, and are not effective for everyone. In sum, for yeast infections, there is no "miracle cure."

If you can, try to avoid the conditions that promote yeast infections. Here are some things you can do to stay infection-free:

- Yeast thrive in warm, moist places. Avoid wearing tight, nylon underwear; wear cotton underwear that allows for the circulation of air. Do not sit around in a wet bathing suit or in sweaty exercise clothes.
- Avoid bingeing on sugary food—yeast thrive on sweets. Curtail alcohol consumption; alcohol is broken down into sugar, which can aggravate a yeast infection.
- Eat yogurt with live cultures. In one study, women with a history of yeast infections who ate two eight-ounce containers of yogurt per day with active acidophilus cultures (so-called good bacteria) had significantly fewer yeast infections than those who did not.
- Get treatment for your sexual partner. In some cases, a yeast infection may be passed by sexual contact. Many gynecologists recommend having your partner treated simultaneously to avoid reinfection.

Resources

THIS SECTION PROVIDES PLACES TO CONTACT FOR FURTHER INFORMATION ON
SOME HEALTH TOPICS OF IMPORTANCE TO WOMEN.

Abortion

Planned Parenthood Federation of
    America
810 Seventh Avenue
New York, NY 10019
212-541-7800

National Women's Health Network
1325 G Street, N.W.
Washington, DC 20005
202-347-1140

**Acquired Immune Deficiency Syndrome
(AIDS)**

National AIDS Hotline
800-342-2437 (English)
800-344-7432 (Spanish)
800-243-7889 (for hearing impaired)

AIDS Clinical Trials Hotline
800-874-2572

National AIDS Clearinghouse
Centers for Disease Control
P.O. Box 6003
Rockville, MD 29849
800-458-5231
800-243-7012 (for hearing impaired)

Aging

National Institute on Aging (NIA)
    Information Center
P.O. Box 8057
Gaithersburg, MD 20898-8057
800-222-2225

Alcohol Abuse

To find support groups, contact:
Alcoholics Anonymous
Check your local telephone direc-
tory under "A" for nearest group.

Al-Anon (for family members of alcoholic)

1327 Broadway
New York, NY 10018
212-302-7240

To find a specialist in treating addictions,
contact:
The American Society of Addiction
    Medicine
12 West 21st Street
New York, NY 10010
212-206-6770

National Council on Alcoholism and
    Drug Dependence
12 West 21st Street, 8th floor
NewYork, NY 10010
800-423-4673

Alzheimer's Disease

Alzheimer's Disease and Related
    Disorders Association
919 North Michigan Avenue

Suite 1000
Chicago, IL 60611
312-335-8700

National Institutes of Health
Building 31
Room 8-A-16
Bethesda, MD 20892

Alzheimer Association
5900Wilshire Boulevard,
    Suite 1710
Los Angeles, CA 90036
213-938-3370

NIA Alzheimer's Disease Education
    and Referral Center (ADEAR)
#NIAC, P.O. Box 8250
Silver Spring, MD 20907-8250
800-438-4380

Arthritis

Arthritis Foundation
1314 Spring Street, NW
Atlanta, GA 30309
800-238-7800

American College of Rheumatology
60 Executive Park South
Atlanta, GA 30329
404-633-3777

National Arthritis and Musculoskeletal
    and Skin Diseases Clearinghouse
    (AMS Clearinghouse)
Box AMS
9000 Rockville Pike
Bethesda, MD 20892
301-495-4484

Asthma

American College of Allergy and
  Immunology Hotline
800-842-7777
Provides information on asthma and allergies

Lung Line
800-222 LUNG or 303-355-LUNG
(Nurses answer your questions on asthma)

Asthma & Allergy Foundation of
  America
1707 North Street, N.W.
Washington, DC 20036
202-966-2222

Blood

American Red Cross National
  Headquarters
17th & D Streets, N.W.
Washington, DC 20006
202-737-8300

Breast Implants

Breast Implant Inquiry
(FDA)
800-532-4440

Food and Drug Administration
Breast Implant Information,HFE-88
5600 Fishers Lane
Rockville, MD 20857
301-443-3170

Cancer

The Susan Koman Foundation

5005 LBJ, Suite 370
Dallas, TX 75244
214-450-1777

National Alliance of Breast Cancer
  Organizations
9 East 37th Street
New York, NY 10016
212-889-0606

American Cancer Society
1599 Clifton Road, NE
Atlanta, GA 30329-4251
404-816-7800

For the latest information on research contact:
The National Cancer Institute
Department of Health and Human
  Services
Building 31, Room 10-A24
9000 Rockville Pike
Bethesda, MD 20892
800-422-6237

Contraception

American College of Obstetrics and
  Gynecologists
409 12th Street, S.W.
Washington, DC 20024-2188
202-638-5577

Planned Parenthood Federation of
  America, Inc.
810 Seventh Avenue
New York, NY 10019
212-541-7800

Dental

American Dental Association

Bureau of Health Education
211 East Chicago Avenue
Chicago, IL 60611
312-440-2500

Diabetes

The American Dietetic Association
216 West Jackson, Suite 800
Chicago, IL 60606
312-899-0040

Eating Disorders

American Anorexia/Bulimia Association
418 East 76th Street, Suite 3B
New York, NY 10021
212-734-1114

Foundation for Education About
    Eating Disorders
5238 Duvall Drive
Bethesda, MD 20816
301-229-6904

Endometriosis

Endometriosis Association
8585 N. 76th Place
Milwaukee, WI 53223
800-992-3636

Eyes

American Optometric Association
243 North Lindbergh Boulevard
St. Louis, MO 63141
314-991-4100

National Eye Institute
National Institutes of Health

Building 31
Bethesda, MD 20893

Exercise

*For information on how to select a sports
club or an exercise trainer, contact:*
American College of Sports Medicine
P.O. Box 1440
Indianapolis, IN 46206
317-637-9200

Eye Care

American Board of Ophthalmology
III Presidential Boulevard, Suite 341
Bala-Cynwyd, PA 19004
215-664-1175

Fibromyalgia

Fibromyalgia Association
P.O. Box 21988
Columbus, OH 43221-0988
614-457-4222

Finding a Doctor

For a list of board-qualified internists,
contact:
American Society of Internal Medicine
1101 Vermont Avenue, N.W.
Washington, DC 20005
202-289-1700

*The American Medical Association will
provide individuals with a physician
profile that lists education and other
credentials for any member.
For a physician profile, contact:*
American Medical Association

535 North Dearborn Street
Chicago, IL 60610
312-645-500

The American Board of Medical Specialists, which oversees certification of specialists in twenty-four different medical specialties, will also check a physician's credentials. For information, call:
800-776-2378

Hair Loss

National Alopecia Areata Foundation
P.O. Box 150760
San Rafael, CA 94915-0760
415-456-4644

Headaches

National Headache Foundation
5252 North Western Avenue
Chicago, IL 60625
800-843-2256

Hearing

The National Research Registry for Hereditary Hearing Loss
Boys Town National Research Hospital
555 North 30th Street
Omaha, NE 68131
402-498-6631 (for hearing impaired)
402-498-6739 (voice)

Heart Disease

American Heart Association
7320 Greenville Avenue
Dallas, TX 75231

214-373-6300
Mended Hearts (For recovering patients and their families)
7320 Greenville Avenue
Dallas, TX 75231
214-373-6300

Hysterectomy

HERS (Hysterectomy Educational Resources & Services)
Bala-Cynwyd, PA 19004
215-667-7757

Incontinence

Continence Restored
785 Park Avenue
New York, NY 10021
212-879-3131

Help for Incontinent People
P.O. Box 544
Union, SC 29379
803-579-7900

American Board of Urology
31700 Telegraph Road, Suite 150
Birmingham, MI 48010
313-646-9720

Infertility

American Fertility Society
2131 Magnolia Avenue, Suite 201
Birmingham, AL 35256
205-978-5000

Lupus

Lupus Foundation of America, Inc.

245

4 Research Place, Suite 180
Rockville, MD 20850-3226
800-558-0121 (for written
    information)
301-670-9292 (for other
    questions)

Mammograms

For information on where to get a mammo-
gram at a facility accredited bythe
American College of Radiology, call:
Cancer Information Service
1-800-4-CANCER

Menopause

North American Menopause Society
2074 Abington Road
Cleveland, OH 44106
216-844-8748

Mental Health

To locate a qualified therapist in your area,
contact:
American Psychological Association
750 First Street, N.E.
Washington, DC
202-336-5700

American Association for Marriage
    and Family Therapy
1100 17th Street, N.W., 10th floor
Washington, D.C. 29936
800-374-2638

National Association of Social
    Workers
750 First Street, N.E.

Washington, DC 20002
202-408-8600

National Mental Health Association
1800 North Kent Street
Arlington, VA 22209
703-684-7722

For information about depression, call:
Depression Awareness, Recognition
and Treatment (D/ART Program)
National Institutes of Mental Health
800-421-4211

Osteoporosis

National Osteoporosis Foundation
1150 17th Street, N.W., Suite 500
Washington, DC 20036
800-223-9994

Calcium Information Center
800-321-2681
(You can hear a recording of the latest med-
ical information and ask questions.)

Plastic Surgery

American Board of Plastic Surgery
7 Penn Center, Suite 400
1635 Market Street
Philadelphia, PA 19103
215-587-9322

American Society of Plastic and
    Reconstructive Surgeons
444 East Algonquin Road
Arlington Heights, IL 60005
800-635-0635

Facial Plastic Surgery Information
   Service
1110 Vermont Avenue, N.W.,
   Suite 220
Washington, DC 20005
800-332-3223

Restless Leg Syndrome

RLS Foundation
304 Glenwood Avenue
Raleigh, NC 27603-1455
919-834-0821

Sjögren's Syndrome

Sjögren's Syndrome Foundation
382 Main Street
Port Washington, NY 11050
516-767-2866

Skin Care

American Board of Dermatology
Henry Ford Hospital
Detroit, MI 48202
313-871-8739

Smoking

For information on how to quit, contact:
The American Lung Association
212-315-8700

Smokenders
800-828-4357

Action on Smoking and Health
2013 H Street, N.W.
Washington, DC 20006
202-659-4310

Vulvar Pain

Vulvar Pain Foundation
910-226-0704

National Vulvodynia Association
301-460-6407

Workplace Health

Environmental Protection Agency
   Indoor Air Pollution Hotline
800-438-4318

Occupational Safety and Health
   Administration (OSHA)
200 Constitution Avenue, N.W.
Washington, DC 20210
202-219-8151

About the Author

MARIANNE LEGATO, M.D. is Director of the new Institute for Gender Specific Medicine at Columbia University College of Physicians and Surgeons. The Institute is devoted to supporting research on women's health issues and to eliminating gender bias in medical research. Dr. Legato is the co-author of THE FEMALE HEART: THE TRUTH ABOUT WOMEN AND CORONARY ARTERY DISEASE, the groundbreaking book that dispelled the myth that heart disease is purely a male problem. She is also one of the nation's leading advocates for women's health.

CAROL COLMAN is a award-winning author and co-author of many popular medical books, including THE FEMALE HEART, THE LUPUS HANDBOOK FOR WOMEN, THE MELA-TONIN MIRACLE, and THE SUPERHOR-MONE PROMISE.